PENGUIN

THE MEMORY CLINIC

TIFFANY CHOW, MD, is a senior clinician-scientist at the Sam and Ida Ross Memory Clinic and Baycrest Health Sciences, where she does clinical research in frontotemporal dementia and Alzheimer's disease. She holds a dual academic appointment as associate professor of neurology and geriatric psychiatry at the University of Toronto. She studied at Stanford University, Rush Medical College, UC San Diego, and UC Los Angeles. She has been a faculty member at UC Los Angeles and the University of Southern California. She lives in Toronto.

THE
MEMORY
CLINIC

Stories of Hope and Healing
for Alzheimer's Patients and Their Families

TIFFANY
CHOW MD

PENGUIN
an imprint of Penguin Canada Books Inc.

Published by the Penguin Group
Penguin Canada Books Inc., 90 Eglinton Avenue East, Suite 700, Toronto, Ontario, Canada M4P 2Y3

Penguin Group (USA) Inc., 375 Hudson Street, New York, New York 10014, U.S.A.
Penguin Books Ltd, 80 Strand, London WC2R 0RL, England
Penguin Ireland, 25 St Stephen's Green, Dublin 2, Ireland (a division of Penguin Books Ltd)
Penguin Group (Australia), 707 Collins Street, Melbourne, Victoria 3008, Australia
(a division of Pearson Australia Group Pty Ltd)
Penguin Books India Pvt Ltd, 11 Community Centre, Panchsheel Park, New Delhi – 110 017, India
Penguin Group (NZ), 67 Apollo Drive, Rosedale, Auckland 0632, New Zealand
(a division of Pearson New Zealand Ltd)
Penguin Books (South Africa) (Pty) Ltd, 24 Sturdee Avenue, Rosebank, Johannesburg 2196,
South Africa

Penguin Books Ltd, Registered Offices: 80 Strand, London WC2R 0RL, England

First published in Viking hardcover by Penguin Canada, 2013
Published in this edition, 2014

1 2 3 4 5 6 7 8 9 10 (WEB)

Manufactured in Canada.

LIBRARY AND ARCHIVES CANADA CATALOGUING IN PUBLICATION

Chow, Tiffany, author
The memory clinic : stories of hope and healing for Alzheimer's
patients and their families / Tiffany Chow, MD.

Originally published: Toronto : Viking, 2013.

Includes bibliographical references and index.

ISBN 978-0-14-318623-6 (pbk.)

1. Alzheimer's disease—Prevention—Popular works. 2. Alzheimer's disease—Treatment—Popular
works. 3. Alzheimer's disease—Patients—Care—Popular works. I. Title.

RC523.2.C56 2014   616.8'31   C2013-906534-2

Visit the Penguin Canada website at **www.penguin.ca**

Special and corporate bulk purchase rates available; please see
www.penguin.ca/corporatesales or call 1-800-810-3104, ext. 2477.

Thanks go to all my teachers great and small,
only a few of whom are mentioned in this book.
I'm grateful to have learned from so many people
who have shared their stories with me
and who have allowed me to become part of their stories.
Your dharma stitches the Hawai'ian quilt of my life together.

CONTENTS

LIFE LESSONS
FROM THE MEMORY CLINIC

I am a senior scientist and behavioral neurologist at the Sam and Ida Ross Memory Clinic at Baycrest in Toronto. I conduct research into dementia as well as treat patients, work which I find both intellectually challenging and spiritually engaging. My practice allows me to help patients and their families at emotionally vulnerable moments. Those experiences are often distressing, sometimes unexpectedly revealing, occasionally funny, and always meaningful. What I learn from these encounters, I parlay into how I manage my own brain-protection strategy.

I resemble many Boomers [in Toronto, we are called Zoomers] who fret not about whether we'll live a long life but rather about how well we will live out our life. I may have a little more concern about retiring into golden years than others do because of my family history of Alzheimer's. Naturally, running a clinic that subspecializes in dementias that start before the age of 65 (early-onset) brings those worries to the forefront.

In 1995, while I was completing my training in neurology in San Diego, I received an unexpected telephone call from my grandfather in Hawai'i. My grandmother Ah Quan had opted not to attend the afternoon funeral of a friend, and Grandpa had gone to pay his respects on their behalf. He returned later in the day to find Ah Quan collapsed on the living room floor. Later, in the emergency room, a CT scan revealed that there had been sudden bleeding into her brain, a hemorrhage. When I arrived at her bedside the next day, I could tell that she was not likely to be conscious enough to feel pain, but the swelling and intracranial trauma had not gone so far as to stop her innate breathing pattern. I did not have to lie to my mother to say that her mother was very deeply asleep. But Ah Quan never woke up. She spent the last month of her life asleep in a rented hospital bed in her living room.

After years of studying dementia through neuroimaging and clinical work, I have only recently recognized Ah Quan's incident as one that is usually caused by Alzheimer's disease. You don't hear about this form of Alzheimer's very often, but one of the effects of Alzheimer's damaging protein deposition in the brain is to weaken the arterial walls until a sudden, large, uncontrolled bleed (think of a collection of blood the size of a grapefruit) ends the person's life. It is called lobar hemorrhage due to amyloid angiopathy, but this stroke-like event does not strike the majority of Alzheimer's patients.

During medical school I had gravitated toward the study of brain disorders that cause behavioral changes, which constitutes the gray zone between neurology and psychiatry. During my residency training in the specialty of neurology, I found a very soft spot in my heart for my elderly patients. Focusing my clinical work and research in the field of dementia brought my career to the rewarding intersection between my scientific interests and my personality type. When I realized, years after setting out on my career path, that Ah Quan had had a form of Alzheimer's disease, it changed my arm's-length relationship to dementia. Like a cliché movie line, I thought, "This time, it's personal."

My family history grants me extra risk for dementia. This book is a summary of what I've learned through my research and from my colleagues about the prevention and management of dementia: Even if we face a family history of Alzheimer's disease and are therefore more vulnerable to dementia, we can prevent its onset or its progression. And it's worth noting that everyone who lives past the age of 65 bears some risk for dementia, regardless of whether their parents or grandparents suffered from it.

Many people use the words *dementia* and *Alzheimer's disease* interchangeably. This is not entirely incorrect, but the two are not synonymous. Dementia is a set of symptoms reported by the patient or family and of signs observable to a doctor's eye, involving a loss of cognitive abilities severe enough to keep an individual from functioning independently. Alzheimer's disease, on the other hand, is one of many possible causes of dementia and is the most common cause in people more than 65 years old. Dementia will occur in more people in more places around the world with each passing year, and many of us already have a friend or family member with dementia. Everyone I meet wants to know what to do to avoid it. While the prospect of brain failure strikes fear into the hearts of many, I have found a natural fit between my outlook on life and what I can offer as a neurologist, counselor, and researcher in this field. Although dementia is caused by some relentless brain disorders, there is meaning—sometimes even joy—to be found through the experience of it, and those moments provide inspiration to those of us who work with dementia every day.

In the early 1980s, the University of California created a program to recruit high school students with potential for academic success. They invited us to participate in selected undergraduate courses, and one really caught my eye: "Medicine, Literature, and Ethics." In that course, I saw how each day in medicine could be wildly different from the last. I learned how patients and their families invite the physician to share in the most intimate aspects of their lives. The physician has the privilege of patients' trusting that she or he can actually help. Despite our efforts, we can't always cure, but I was dazzled by the opportunity to make such a direct difference to people.

Now, as a specialist in cognitive impairment, I care not only for the patients but also for their caregiver family members and close friends. This rounds out a holistic, multifaceted approach to the illness. A professional team can really help caregivers to understand and appreciate the special roles they are playing in the face of an incurable illness.

Leading families through the difficult step of accepting a diagnosis of dementia or Alzheimer's and the subsequent stages of intervention and adaptation has granted me a privileged view of life's changes. It has shown me that dementia can be considered as part of a long series of life changes. Moreover, that view of inevitable changes is consistent with the tenets of Buddhism, and, indeed, has allowed me to understand some of its practices more deeply. Practicing what are known as the

"Four Intentions" from Buddhism—equanimity, compassion, kindness, and joy—has allowed me to connect meaningfully with the families in our clinic. And that practice has enriched my personal life immeasurably, staving off burnout and enabling me to remain flexible and open to where my research needs to go to make a difference.

Likewise, my job has been made easier and more fulfilling by imparting that approach to caregivers, both family members and those on the professional health care team. The aim is to help them to help themselves, and to be of more assistance to the patient. Even if we can't cure the dementia, we can model for caregivers how to provide care. My former professor in the Emergency Department at the University of California, San Diego, Dr. Tom Neuman, urged us to remember that, "The patient is always having a worse day than you." Over time, though, I've learned that sometimes I am having a worse day than the patient. Mastering the role of caregiver begins with caring for self, extending loving kindness to oneself. It means taking stock of one's own situation and asking: "Do I feel safe? Do I feel loved? Do I feel healthy?" The answer may reveal that a caregiver has sacrificed his or her own health to the needs of the patient. "Do I feel happy?" If an individual's happiness is related solely to being a good caregiver, it takes a major shift in thinking to find a new definition of happiness. "Am I living with ease? Am I allowed to, as a caregiver?"

Dharma refers to the philosophical and spiritual teachings of learned Buddhists. One of my favorite dharma teachers, Sharon Salzberg, challenges her audiences of health professionals to look after themselves, too. "If I said spending 20 minutes a day on a particular activity would significantly help one of your friends, how many of you would do it? Without skipping a beat, her listeners usually all raise their hands. Then comes the kicker: "So why is it so hard for us to spend 20 minutes a day meditating or exercising or slowing down to take care of our*selves*?" Extending loving kindness toward oneself is one of the most vital survival tips I can pass on to caregivers. It trumps teaching them how to pronounce the generic names of medications.

A doctor I once met asked me if I knew how to translate the Latin word *equanimitas* into a medical setting. To him, it meant, "The physician must treat all things the same, not allowing emotion to rule." As an eager young student inspired by patients' stories, I thought, "Oh dear, I'm not going to be good at that." But in retrospect, I agree with the man. If compassion is not informed by wisdom and equanimity, one can act foolishly and ineffectively. I have learned that equanimity is not indifference; rather it is the practice of compassion without picking favorites and also without prejudice against those things we fear. There are, on the one hand, intentions, and there are, on the other, skills to help us execute those intentions. When I applied to medical school, I knew I had good intentions, and I was hoping to learn skills to implement those intentions. Medical school teaches us how to use instruments, chemistry, biology, genetics, and pharmacology to make an impact on a patient's life. But the kind of skill referred to in Buddhist teachings helps to ensure that the impact is positive for both the giver and the recipient of the act. As I continue my practice, I seek ways to balance my own life and to provide compassionate care to patients and their families.

1

A VISIT TO THE CLINIC

People make a lot of nervous jokes about "senior moments." My parents and their friends ask anxiously if having lost track of their car in the parking lot at the shopping mall means that they are getting Alzheimer's disease. "I think I'm losing it" nowadays indicates fear of the initial stage of a dementia, instead of a problem with an anger management issue or an impending nervous breakdown. An increasing number of patients in memory clinics can be considered "the worried well." These individuals are highly motivated to follow up on the history of Alzheimer's disease in a parent or grandparent and seek advice as to how to avoid the dementia, if possible.

Laura is in her fifties. Her father died in his late fifties of an odd, quickly progressing illness, which made him at first irresponsible and disorganized, then rapidly incapable of taking care of himself. To add to the tragedy of this early-onset illness (dementia more typically strikes those over 65 years old), doctors weren't sure of the diagnosis. His genetic test results were negative for Huntington's disease (the movement disorder with cognitive and psychiatric symptoms that killed singer-songwriter Woody Guthrie). Two years ago, Laura's older brother Glen was diagnosed at my clinic with Alzheimer's disease, at the age of 53. Speaking with their mother, I learned that Glen likely had the same rapidly progressing dementia as his father.

Laura and her husband run a landscaping business. They've been together since they met, managing their crew and getting their hands dirty with yard work. During cold Toronto winters, they clear snow out of driveways and off of sidewalks. They look like they could be in their thirties, despite drinking more alcohol and smoking more cigarettes than they should. They are the best of business partners and friends. Laura's mother has been fearful that Laura is starting to have symptoms that will eventually disrupt this happy life, so she asked us to invite Bill and Laura to come in for an evaluation shortly after Glen was diagnosed. It has taken Bill and Laura a year to make that appointment.

They arrive at Baycrest, a complex designed for geriatric care at the north end of Toronto, where my clinic operates. Baycrest offers a huge 600-bed nursing home; a hospital for those residents who need acute care and rehabilitation; a retirement home for folks enjoying better health; day programs; and multiple ambulatory care clinics for intersection with hearing specialists, geriatric medicine, physiotherapy, occupational therapy, mobility, geriatric psychiatry, family medicine, and my own subspecialty, behavioral neurology. The architects made sure that all buildings have ramped access, grab rails on all the walls, large elevator buttons for those with visual impairment, and open gathering places for those in wheelchairs and accompanying persons. This center for geriatric care has been an innovative leader in the field, and I was recruited to do both research and clinical care in dementia, in affiliation with the other excellent health care centers that gather under the academic umbrella of the University of Toronto.

My research office is on the ninth floor of the building, adjacent to the original Jewish Home for the Aged that over the decades burgeoned into this one-stop geriatric center. Just down the hall are major players in the scientific study of memory, recognized internationally for their groundbreaking and seminal work in correlating specific aspects of memory to small brain regions and theorizing on what role consciousness plays in effective memory function. Testing rooms where young research assistants carry out the scientists' experiments are located downstairs. The clinic where I see patients in their fifties and sixties with early-onset dementia is on the sixth floor, conveniently close by so that I can use the stairwell between my two offices as needed. Often my sixth-floor patients are keen to participate in our research, so they get to know both the clinic area and the testing rooms.

Bill and Laura arrive at the sixth-floor Memory Clinic to meet me and my nurse Mindy for their first appointment. They are both very much aware of what happened to Laura's father and brother, and appearing in my clinic to have this evaluation is an important step in accepting that there is a family history placing Laura at risk for a similar set of problems. It was tempting for them to believe that the recent difference in function was related to menopause, since Laura had just experienced that life change. But they both seem to know that she is starting to have the family's illness.

Mindy starts by running through our checklist of possible symptoms of dementia, beginning with memory but not stopping there. People with dementia develop a constellation of impairments that can affect concentration, mathematical calculations, way-finding, motivation level, and temper. Laura and Bill have noticed that Laura has become increasingly disorganized, although she is reluctant to admit it. The nurse makes notes on when each of the cognitive changes started (there were no behavioral changes). Now that he's being asked, Bill realizes that for the last year he has gradually increased assisting with or double-checking on her tasks.

Laura has been healthy enough not to have to take any medications. She has not been depressed (which is often a cause of slight memory problems and decreased concentration in this age group). She has not had any significant head traumas during her lifetime. She has barely had to see a physician at all during her life. The nurse relays this summary of the information to me while Bill and Laura wait for the next part of the evaluation in our waiting room, no doubt daunted by the advanced age of the other patients who have come to see my colleagues in the clinic. Those patients are 76 and up, using a walker or accompanied by one family member and one young, typically Filipina or Caribbean hired personal support worker. Mindy reminds me of the significant family history, and we take a mutual deep breath to acknowledge the gravity of the situation. No one wishes dementia on anyone, and we feel for Laura and Glen's mother, who will have seen at least three of her loved ones pass through this illness.

I bring Laura into my office for testing. I don't bring significant others into the room for this part of the evaluation unless I need them to translate our questions. Family members have usually been helping patients with dementia to answer questions for a year or two before they come to see me, and it's hard to stifle this newly acquired habit. When family members coach too much, I have to remind them that, in this place, I do need to see exactly where the patient's strengths and weaknesses lie. When we all recall that everyone has strengths and weaknesses, my role becomes more like a solicitous service provider and less like a Grand Inquisitor.

The testing starts with a long counting backward task that lets us know about the integrity of calculations and also indicates how long someone can stick to the same task, no matter how boring. Laura is a bit nervous about what we might find, and I apologize for making her feel uncomfortable, encouraging her wherever she answers correctly. Laura has some difficulty with every aspect of the testing. We frequently find that there are more areas of impairment than families were aware of.

We ask patients about the date, the season of the year, and if they know exactly where we are (what building, what city), and this is often not a problem for a patient early in illness. This provides me an opportunity to give some encouragement. Naming objects that I show them (*shoe*, *heel*, *thumb*) can be difficult for patients with Alzheimer's disease, and Laura cannot perform perfectly at this. She has difficulty remembering a short frequently used word list (*cat*, *apple*, *table*). This is something we see typically among the elderly who have Alzheimer's disease.

She can make a good copy of most figures (such as a cube, or two pentagons that overlap at one corner). That might be a resilient talent because of the nature of her and Bill's landscaping work. They need to plant things in the right places, translating from diagrams to actual yard space.

Next are tasks that can detect whether a patient's mind gets trapped in purposeless repetition of a movement and language abilities. These abilities are still intact for Laura. She is able to switch tasks easily and to express herself clearly when asked questions, but she doesn't offer much spontaneous speech, which might be within the usual range for her quiet, practical personality.

The physical portion of the examination is much easier for both doctor and patient in early-onset dementia cases. These patients, by dint of their age, are typically still as quick and strong as I am, and are free of arthritic disability or cardiac problems that can cause fatigue. A neurologist checks the patient's muscular strength, coordination, and reflexes, and Laura's physical condition is perfect. She feels competent on this type of testing. I am happy for another opportunity to give her good feedback instead of remaining discreetly silent. But by my mental calculations, Laura's likelihood of dying from Alzheimer's disease within the next 10 years is high.

At the end of the visit, we have to confirm aloud that Laura is starting to have the same symptoms as her brother Glen. We discuss whether things will change as quickly for her as they had for him. Bill and Laura hold hands tightly during this talk. They are able to hear me, they aren't surprised, and Bill sums up their response by saying, "Well, things are good now, and we'll just get through this together as it comes." I tell them about available medication, and we agree to start Laura on the same medication that had seemed to help Glen a little bit. There are three medications currently available from the same drug class to treat (but not cure) Alzheimer's disease, and Glen had only tolerated one of them well.

When Mindy and I offer caregiver support groups and written materials on Alzheimer's disease to them, Bill demurs. While we are hopeful that we can intervene early and regularly to support Bill, he seems resistant, and we respect whatever time he might need to adjust to the pronouncement of the diagnosis. On parting, Bill and Laura agree that minimizing, or better yet, stopping the alcohol intake and smoking might help her optimize brain function.

We see them again about six months later. They've succeeded in eliminating alcohol but smoking is still a challenge. Laura seems the same as on the first visit, and we hypothesize that the medication is helping to stabilize her. Bill doesn't want to talk much about future planning, and Laura seems nervous about being in a doctor's office, although she is cooperative with the abbreviated testing I do in visits that come after that first three-hour appointment.

The following year, Bill shares with us his frustration that Laura is becoming a liability at work, without insight as to how she is creating confusion and problems with their staff and work orders. He has begun to work with their close-knit staff to make sure she is always under supervision and that she only goes onsite for jobs when appropriate. On a timeline that Bill has determined, we have enrolled Laura in a day program since she has developed a tendency to wander (just because you can't work at a job doesn't mean you don't seek some sort of stimulation), and most recently, Laura has some personal support workers to spend the daytime with her.

Bill has been especially impressive in his flexibility and adaptation to a shifting situation. Although he didn't necessarily have to, he has stopped smoking, which has helped to reinforce

Laura's smoking cessation. Shortly after he admitted that Laura couldn't function at work anymore, he realized that he could easily sell their successful landscaping business. The new owners hired him, and life was suddenly easier because he had less responsibility at work. With more time and energy for non-work activities, he could spend more quality time with Laura. No one knows Laura better than he, and he is able to make her feel safe and laugh at the drop of a hat. An old Swedish proverb advises, "Love me when I least deserve it, because that's when I really need it." He also spends time visiting Glen, relieving the family's unaffected sibling, Gary, from some of his caregiving duties.

Laura has lost the ability to generate words and sentences on her own. On their last visit to my office, she responds to conversation by repeating the speaker's tone of voice and length of phrase, but with gibberish sounds. She still understands context and laughs at whatever humor Bill and I bring into the conversation. She is still strong but a little jittery sitting in her seat—she can't understand what I'm asking her to do when I ask her to move her hands in ways to demonstrate whether her coordination and aim are true, but she can imitate what I do, so the examination takes on a feeling of play.

Bill answers honestly about how well or poorly she's doing. He is nothing but pleasant and affectionate with her; she leans into him whenever he's nearby. When she can't see him, he indicates with his eyes that things are not easy at home: She has developed urinary incontinence when she is taking too much of a medication that keeps her from being too restless. I do my best to acknowledge that look with a nodding, slow blink to indicate I understand and wish it weren't so. We opt for less medication, better bladder control, and maybe more restlessness. But I can tell she's slowing down because two years ago she used to try to get up to leave my office every five minutes, and now she sits until we all stand up to signify that the visit is coming to a close.

Bill has maintained his attitude that they will get through it together. At the end of this most recent visit, Laura becomes confused as the two of them stand at my receptionist's window, laughing somewhat hysterically as a non-verbal commentary. Bill turns her to face him, picks her up off the ground in his burly arms, and she gleefully wraps her arms and legs around him, instantly reassured. This is the moment I work for. We should all be so lucky as to have such loving companionship, even when it is complicated by an illness like dementia. And in the absence of a cure for dementia, my goal is to help families have more of those joyful, connecting moments. To experience joy and love does not require perfect cognitive function.

Specifically, dementia is diagnosed when two or more cognitive domains have become significantly impaired. If someone has memory loss but only memory loss, even if it is severe, that person may be diagnosed as amnestic but not necessarily as having a dementia. I often tell medical students that after a long night of sleep deprivation, we might not be able to remember to pick up some items at the grocery store on the way home and we might be a little grouchy, but these are mild impairments and easily remedied by a break, so they don't qualify us for dementia.

Doctors and rocket scientists are not immune to Alzheimer's disease, but people with high levels of education can be tough to test adequately with our standard battery. While I was working in

Los Angeles, I met an aeronautics engineer who admitted that he fit the description of "rocket scientist." It was nearly impossible for me to ask Gene questions that he couldn't answer correctly (I have never been that sharp at chemistry and calculus). He was convinced, however, that he wasn't as capable of multitasking recently and was processing information more slowly. Gene scored well above normal ranges of function, but the important part was his own report of decline. A familiar example would be to note that your computer is taking longer to perform tasks— it's just slower, not crashing, and the email still gets sent to the right destination, but you know it used to be more efficient. It's especially disquieting to these supernormal patients to be told not to worry because they're "still ahead of the curve." The machinery is not working like it used to, and since the brain is not replaceable or transplantable, the neurologist needs to help such a patient understand whether this is expected aging or premature, abnormal loss of function.

After assessing Gene for personality changes or impairment in social skills, I consulted our team neuropsychologist to give him the more difficult tests in the other cognitive domains: memory, executive function, calculations, language, and visuo-spatial ability.

Loss of independence is a key component in deciding whether a person meets criteria for dementia. This is a way to gauge severity of cognitive impairment on a person-by-person basis. Although Gene was vividly aware that he was losing strength of mind, he was still able to complete his work without supervision and to navigate the world for errands and social interactions, so we told him he had Mild Cognitive Impairment, which sometimes develops into dementia. We follow patients with Mild Cognitive Impairment annually—memory will worsen fairly quickly in approximately 20% of them over the first year after diagnosis, but not all will convert to Alzheimer's disease.

Alternatively, patients with a dementia often minimize their difficulties or are unaware of them, hence we like to ask friends or family for confirmation of a patient's retained abilities. Activities of daily living are split into two categories: instrumental and basic. Instrumental activities of daily living are those things that allow your interactions with the outside world, such as keeping appointments or paying your bills. Basic activities of daily living have to do with personal hygiene, such as bathing or dressing.

A physician relies heavily on corroborated reports of independence in activities of daily living. I hear frequently in response to our set questionnaire that a male patient does not participate in household chores. The very important follow-up question is whether he ever helped around the house. For today's elders, the man's place was not in the kitchen, so we need to ask about any changes to activities he pursued during his mid-life.

Hallie was described by her daughter Samantha as having always been a "flighty artist." The mother had taken to abdicating roles she was no longer interested in playing, quickly responding, "I don't know" to all questions. Samantha wondered whether her mother was just being a little more of a diva than usual or if she was beginning to have a dementia.

Given the willfulness of Samantha's mother, it would be hard to determine her level of cognitive function through the usual round of mental status testing ("What day is it? What floor of the building are we on?"). Those kinds of tests are only valid when the patient is putting full effort into the session. In Hallie's case, it was better to try a more organic approach. I asked Samantha if her mother, who had been a painter all her life, was still painting. Was she able to mix her own paints? Could she relate the brush to the canvas meaningfully? Did she paint in the same style as before? Samantha replied that her mother had switched from the medium of oil paints to making sketches. The sketches were good. A change in medium within a lifelong skill set is not cause for alarm—perhaps her mother was enjoying a change in her mode of expression! And basic activities of daily living were still intact. So far, there wasn't much cause for alarm. We advised Samantha to watch closely for a clearer sign of functional loss in her mum. Then it might be easier to tell what's going on.

Perhaps it will turn out to have been a brief depression. Mood disorders are quite common within the geriatric population. Sometimes the obstinacy as reported by Samantha is a symptom of depression or a reaction to stressful change or even chronic pain.

People do change over time. Much of the challenge we face in diagnosing dementia lies in exploring whether the degree of change observed has gone outside the range of typical human adaptation to other aspects of long life, such as retirement or surviving good friends and loved ones.

2

CAUSES OF DEMENTIA

There are many ways in which a person can come to a diagnosis of dementia. For example, a major head injury from a car accident followed years later by a stroke can lead to acquired cognitive impairment in two or more domains, depending on the location of the injuries. And those two insults to the brain could occur in a person of any age, not just in an elderly person.

Of the many causes of dementia in people over the age of 45, Alzheimer's disease is the most commonly occurring. That is likely why you've heard so much about it. In the 1990s, the most common cause of dementia among the younger population was human immunodeficiency virus, or HIV. Happily, better antiviral medications have markedly decreased the number of HIV-positive patients who experience that severe a degree of cognitive impairment.

The primary feature of Alzheimer's disease is memory loss, but other cognitive domains are affected. From the executive function domain, people early in Alzheimer's disease may notice that they are less able to multitask successfully. Or they may not be able to perform the calculations necessary to understand whether refinancing a mortgage helps or hurts the household budget.

From the language domain, the most common early complaint of Alzheimer's disease patients is that they have difficulty finding the word that they want to use in conversation. This usually starts with difficulty finding a word that is not frequently used, such as *hem*. Words more frequently used in daily conversation, such as *dress*, may not be as difficult to retrieve until later in the illness.

Difficulty with visuospatial function refers to not being able to find your car at the shopping mall or not being able to orient yourself to a new airport despite adequate signage. Sometimes this particular deficit hasn't been noted by family, yet it becomes apparent when the patient comes into the clinic for testing.

Changes in personality or social skills may come only later in the course of Alzheimer's disease. A mild case of dementia may keep you from being able to manage your finances by yourself but allow you to appear on time and appropriately dressed for social events. Late in dementia, however, most patients have lost motivation and have withdrawn from most activities. Other common types of dementia among persons over 45 years old include dementia with Lewy bodies, frontotemporal dementia, and vascular cognitive impairment.

Dementia with Lewy bodies (DLB) is most easily understood as a combination of Alzheimer's disease and Parkinson's disease. These patients generally experience the start of memory loss and the physical rigidity of Parkinson's disease within the first two years of illness. Having both types of problems at once can create confusion for the family if physicians disagree on the diagnosis. The decline in memory and other cognitive domains may proceed more quickly than the signs of halting Parkinsonian movement or vice versa. In early stages of the illness these patients will have more difficulty with visuospatial function than patients with Alzheimer's disease.

Parkinson's disease itself can lead to a different form of dementia, usually only after the patient has had Parkinson's disease for approximately a decade. In these cases, patients lose executive function, which then can lead to difficulty encoding new information if the patient develops an attention deficit. Therefore the dementia in late Parkinson's disease can look like memory loss on the surface but has more to do with inattentiveness and inability to juggle information for quick and facile responses. Dementia caused by chronic Parkinson's disease also does not show the early visuospatial impairments appreciated in DLB.

Fascinatingly, sometimes people sustain large brain injuries without manifesting significant or lasting cognitive impairment. Andy went to work on a day that seemed like any other until he developed the worst headache of his life. Shortly after mentioning it aloud, he fell to the ground. Co-workers were stunned that someone in his thirties could be felled so easily, but he had fallen into a coma due to a bloody hemorrhage into his brain. When he recovered a few months later, he was able to return to his job *scheduling moon rocket launches for NASA*. On hearing this history after Andy had retired, I thought, "Gee, must not have been that large a lesion." But when I placed Andy's brain scans on the light board, a gaping hole in the right side of his brain taunted me. Forty years after his stroke, I could plainly see that the man was missing most of his right frontal lobe, and that it had been missing since that coma. Yet he had enjoyed an on-schedule retirement, surviving to the point where, 40 years after the coma, he needed an evaluation for new memory loss. Not all brain injury causes dementia. And having had a major brain trauma does not prevent you from developing a late-life dementia unless it ends your life. It had taken the onset of Alzheimer's disease to make this man less than normal to his colleagues and family, not a severe loss of tissue from the largest lobe of his brain!

One thing that sets Alzheimer's disease apart from other causes of dementia is the type of abnormal protein collection that accumulates in the brain of the patient. Alzheimer's disease in almost all cases is related to a combination of *amyloid plaques* and *neurofibrillary tangles*.

The amyloid plaques have gotten more attention from researchers than the neurofibrillary tangles in the last decade, because some genetic mutations linked the development of Alzheimer's disease to factors that increase the production of *beta-amyloid*, the form of amyloid protein that clumps together to make the plaques. Ordinarily, the brain and other cells of the body are making amyloid that is in a usable form. However, at a certain point (possibly both genetically and environmentally determined), the same machinery that once produced the normally occurring form of amyloid also begins to extrude the beta form, which is longer and stickier. These molecules of beta-amyloid at first form little pieces called oligomers, which themselves wind into strands called fibrils, and then these fibrils stick together to form the plaques. The leading theory about amyloid has been that the amyloid plaques cause neuronal dysfunction and then the symptoms of Alzheimer's disease. There are recent clues that the beta-amyloid fibrils interfere with the cell membrane surface in ways that prevent that cell from absorbing what it needs from its surroundings (which it normally does in a process called *endocytosis*). Others have suggested that these amyloid plaques themselves are a reaction to something else, such as the formation of neurofibrillary tangles.

Neurofibrillary tangles are made up of a protein called tau, which becomes sticky when a phosphorus group is added to the structure. Sticky amyloid forms plaques and sticky tau forms tangles that can be seen within neurons. Something causes the lifelong production of these two otherwise vital proteins to "go rogue."

Chemically speaking, another change characterizing Alzheimer's disease is the loss of the brain's ability to manufacture acetylcholine. When present, plaque and tangle formations appear in the areas of the brain that produce acetylcholine, causing a reduction and eventual crisis in acetylcholine levels. Most of the medications approved for treatment of Alzheimer's disease address this cholinergic deficit.

Frontotemporal dementia is the type of dementia that got me most interested in pursuing research. As opposed to affecting the rear half of the brain, as does Alzheimer's disease or DLB, frontotemporal dementia has a predilection for the front half. Those areas of the brain help us to modulate our behavior and create our own internal reality checks about how we are doing socially. Without these regions of the brain working at their best, we can easily alienate family members, friends, and co-workers.

I can easily see myself as the same person regardless of whether my memory is fantastic or poor, because I still enjoy my same activities, likes, and dislikes. Frontotemporal dementia can entirely destroy a person's temper, ability to sustain friendships, and enjoyment of former social activities or hobbies. Motivation to do both instrumental and basic activities of daily living is often affected, in a very subtle way at first, but then progressing rapidly over time. This dementia would alter your very personality, making you into a stranger among those who have known you best.

One afternoon, a man was accompanied to our clinic by his wife and his elderly mother. If this had been the usual case, my patient would have been the elderly mother; the man, her number one son; and the woman, the daughter-in-law and the primary caregiver for the mother. Instead, the 50-year-old man was the patient. The couple had four sons ranging in age from 10 to 16. The first symptoms of Richard's dementia were drastic changes in his temper and fathering skills. Whereas he had been very close to his sons, very supportive, affectionate, and a great hockey dad, for the past year, he had been verbally abusive and frightened the family with his outbursts. He had broken things around the home. And at work he was unable to function productively, so he had lost his job, leaving his wife as the family's sole breadwinner.

Richard's mother sat quietly and sadly in the room with us until we got to the part of the interview in which I asked if anyone in the family had had similar symptoms in the past. The somber mood in the room descended a few more notches.

At this point, the mother described in English with a very thick Cantonese accent that Richard's father had had the very same symptoms and had died after a few years of illness at 50, Richard's current age. Richard's wife, Lily, added that Richard had been the primary caregiver for his father and had even wondered aloud at the time whether he would suffer the same fate. Richard, meanwhile, was quieter than all of them but might answer with a few words when directly addressed.

Once his mother started to speak, it seemed she could not stop. She said that she would spend as many days of the week away from her own home to supervise Richard as she could, but she was "an old lady" and had problems of her own. She was, of course, concerned about his welfare, but she was overwhelmed by the realization that she would survive her son the way she had her husband, and concerned about the rest of her children and grandchildren. She seemed to be avoiding a discussion about his disease and its possible heritability by launching into her own laundry list of medical ailments.

My upbringing taught me to respect my elders. That trait, especially with this Chinese family, was hampering my ability to learn more about Richard. It was hard to interrupt his mother and get back to the matter at hand. None of us really wanted to talk about how quickly this illness would progress, given Richard's father's pattern. No one wanted to acknowledge that each of those four sons, not all of whom had reached their teens yet, was at risk to develop what their father and grandfather had. Hearing and accepting the diagnosis would require some sensitive discussion among many more people than just the patient and one caregiver.

After the initial interview, I asked Richard's mother and

Lily to leave the room so that I could test Richard's memory and other cognitive skills. I usually follow that with a physical exam to look for problems with coordination, eye movements, and smoothness of muscle movement, which might provide clues about the underlying diagnosis. As the door shut behind the ladies, I wondered if Richard and I would be able to have much meaningful communication, given that he had been so quiet and withdrawn during the interview. Due to his illness, at first Richard looked at me, unblinking, for long enough that I needed to turn my gaze away. He did seem to understand the context of the visit, though, which prompted me to ask if he thought he might have the same thing his father had. At that, his eyes instantly welled up with tears and he nodded up and down in terrified agreement. My heart already felt full from the interview, and his obvious awareness was very difficult. We just sat there for a minute, then instead of reining in his emotions to continue with the exam, he sobbed, "I'm so sorry!" He had not wanted any of this: to become someone alien to his sons; to be a burden to his mother, who was still grieving the loss of her husband; and to be a burden to his young family. And he, of all people, knew how much of a burden he would become and how quickly. I wished for him a more immediate loss of insight. As dreaded, he did horribly on cognitive testing, which indicated that the disease was indeed fast-moving. And he had signs of rigidity on one side of his body already.

After I finished the physical exam, Lily and Richard's mother rejoined us. I have learned that the only way for me to serve a family at this level of crisis is to drop the typical doctor's agenda of scribbling out a prescription and sending the family back to the receptionist to book their next appointment. Instead they need me to be as entirely present as possible. It's best when I abandon all pretense of being able to control the illness or the family's ability to cope with it, and instead acknowledge how much suffering there is in the room.

This is different from what we are taught in popular culture. It's easy to get wrapped up in television's "House"-type ideal of the doctor: cocky enough to discourage resistance, and able to use a small amount of information about the patient to carry out a high-speed mental search of medical know-how to make a crack diagnosis and then rattle off the tried-and-true plan for cure—much to the amazement of everyone in the room. But that doesn't happen in the world of dementia.

The family already knew from watching Richard's father that this was a serious illness that would shorten his life considerably. I did not have to tell them that we had no cure for it, but they needed to hear it from me, in order for it to erupt into reality so that they could begin to act on the news. Richard's mother again retreated to a focus on her own medical conditions. I understood better why this was such an unbelievably difficult situation for her after Lily's parting comment to me: She thought that Richard's younger sister should come in for an evaluation also.

I immediately went to Mindy's office to debrief. I usually book enough time to run down to my nurse's office for us to discuss our new cases. Sometimes we're so overwhelmed by the story as it unfolds that we can't think clearly until after the family has left the clinic. Mindy and I don't waste much time ranting about Fate. We mutually acknowledge how sad the story is, and then we double-check whether there's anything else we can offer or teach. Then, the show must go on. Other patients await us.

In this case, she acknowledged that Richard was a young patient, but most of my patients are young at the early-onset dementia clinic. She waited to hear my explanation of why I was so affected. I choked out that Richard could have been my brother. Since my relatives live in Los Angeles and Honolulu, it is easy for my Toronto friends not to have them on their radar. Suddenly Mindy understood perfectly well that this case was way too close to home for me.

In addition to the marked behavioral changes, patients with frontotemporal dementia lose executive function, becoming very distractible and disorganized. The fact that this particular dementia has an early onset, tending to strike when patients are middle-aged as opposed to in their late seventies, leads to a great deal of diagnostic confusion. The most frequent first diagnoses are "mid-life crisis," "depression," "recurrence of attention deficit disorder from childhood," or "new substance abuse." Frontotemporal dementia is particularly insidious because it strikes at such an important time in the adult lifespan. Patients are disrupted from their work lives and parenting. I've been so moved by the courage and generosity of the children of my patients who have become terrific caregivers that we created a website to help support them through the challenges they face as they grow up.

The discovery of abnormal proteins in the brains of frontotemporal dementia patients has been the big news in dementia research from 2008 to 2012. Although tau is a component in the neurofibrillary tangles of Alzheimer's disease, a different but also sticky form of tau is responsible for the abnormality in a large proportion of frontotemporal dementia cases. More recently, even more frontotemporal dementia cases were linked to a protein called TDP-43, and some of these cases revealed a genetic mutation involving a protein called progranulin. Interestingly, this mutation does not lead to collections of progranulin in the brain. Progranulin apparently helps to control how TDP-43 is formed, and when the genetic mutation causes insufficient progranulin manufacture, the TDP-43 cannot be processed normally. The shortened TDP-43 then gets delivered mistakenly to the center of the neuron, where it clumps into stress granules. They're called stress granules because they form in response to chemical cell stressors, not personal stressors. Because these stress granules grab onto the cell's RNA (a middleman for the translation of DNA into actual protein), they effectively set off a cascade of brain-destroying processes, possibly as seen in the other types of dementia with abnormal protein collections. The homework for researchers is to discover why TDP-43 is not exclusive to frontotemporal dementia—it is present in Alzheimer's disease and DLB as well. This could indicate a final common insult to the brain or a final brain distress signal in response to neurode-generative disease.

A different cause of dementia is interrupted blood flow to the brain. This is also known as stroke causing dementia, vascular cognitive impairment, or vascular dementia. A wide range of stroke types are implicated. Some individuals sustain chronic, progressive "clogs" in the smallest bore plumbing, which leads to dysfunction of the white matter deep in the brain. (Think of small brown patches on a lawn that has chronic, grainy mineral deposits clogging its sprinklers.) Others suffer serial blockages of medium-sized arteries, which is shown by a stepwise decline in function. Others may meet criteria for vascular dementia after just two large strokes.

The cognitive domains affected in vascular cognitive impairment or dementia correlate with the areas hit by the stroke. Physicians feel most certain about this diagnosis when we can see the strokes on the CT or MRI scan and can correlate them in time to the reported onset of loss of functions for those regions. For example, "Dad has been gradually more distractible and unable to complete woodworking projects for the last two to four years" might go with a scan that shows multiple splotches in the white matter. If, a year later, this difficulty with attention has worsened and there has been a sudden loss of language comprehension, we would expect to see more splotches or even a confluence of the white-matter splotches plus a new area of tissue damage in the temporal lobe on a second MRI scan. If this patient were no longer able to perform his instrumental activities of daily living following that stroke, he would meet criteria for vascular dementia. Andy, the NASA retiree, only had the one large, old stroke on his MRI, removing vascular cognitive impairment from the list of possible dementia causes.

Rehabilitation specialists seek ways to restore function after stroke. Regaining cognition can be trickier than regaining movement and strength, but it remains within the realm of possibility if the blockage of blood flow does not persist too long or over too large a region of the brain. To prevent progression from mild vascular cognitive impairment to dementia, patients' stroke risk factors—smoking, high blood pressure, and diabetes—must be managed carefully.

Regardless of the cause, no one wants to get dementia and no one wishes it upon anyone else. Yet dementia is a mushrooming health care priority.

3

DEFENSES AGAINST DEMENTIA

When it comes to defenses against dementia, most researchers argue that there is such a thing as "cognitive reserve"—a set of conditions that can compensate for and minimize symptoms. Your cognitive reserve can be your shield. One set of findings that has raised optimism among Alzheimer's disease researchers, and especially for me, is that there are quite a few individuals who have Alzheimer's disease plaques and neurofibrillary tangles in their brains at the time of death, yet those same people have not shown significant cognitive impairment that resembles Alzheimer's disease.

Autopsy data show that individuals with higher educational levels can compensate for Alzheimer's disease pathology better than patients with a lower educational level. A person with only elementary school level achievement will therefore be likely to need help with daily functions even when there is a low level of plaques and tangles present in the brain; on the other hand, someone with a high school educational level or higher seems to show only negligible memory loss or even no symptoms at all, despite having acquired the same mild stage of microscopic Alzheimer's changes to the brain.

I'll never forget an amazing case that presented itself at the University of California, Los Angeles. A family practitioner was earning some post-retirement "pin money" by serving as the physician for a men's correctional facility. He suddenly experienced a rapid decline in cognitive function and his whole body jerked when he was startled by a noise. Those foreboding symptoms indicated he had Creutzfeldt–Jakob disease, a fairly rare cause of dementia that leads to the patient's demise in fewer than two years. Later, an autopsy revealed that he had already harbored enough plaques and tangles to qualify for a diagnosis of Alzheimer's disease, but it had taken the unfortunate addition of a *second* neurological disorder for him to show cognitive difficulty.

This means that if you or I were to accumulate amyloid plaques and neurofibrillary tangles due to genetic programming beyond our control, we might be able to compensate for those brain changes. Until we know how to eradicate amyloid plaques or neurofibrillary tangles that have already formed, we will seek those activities or medications that will allow us to compensate for their presence. This is where the concept of education level as a means of bolstering one's cognitive reserve comes in.

The intellectual challenge of completing higher education is said to develop brain circuitry to back up the areas that commonly conduct the business of remembering, problem solving, and communication. With a rich network of collateral circuits, then, even if a person has the abnormal proteins of Alzheimer's disease accumulating in her brain, she has more compensatory capacity to prevent outwardly noticeable cognitive impairment. This principle may hold true for non-Alzheimer's dementias, as well.

Cognitive reserve—the accumulation of brain benefits from innate intelligence and advanced education—can make the difference in whether two individuals at the same stage of abnormal protein deposition are equally disabled by it. (Cognitive reserve has also been referred to as *cerebral reserve* in the past.)

My grandmother set a good example of how to build and maintain cognitive reserve over a lifespan. Ah Quan was born in Honolulu, Hawai'i, in 1906, the eldest of 11 children. Ah Quan's father had found employment as a cook for the Greens, a missionary family descended from Reverend Jonathan Green. Reverend Green came in the third American wave to what were called the Sandwich Isles (prior to Hawai'i) on the *Parthian* in 1828. He soon parted ways with that original missionary company when he became concerned about their support for slavery. One of the good reverend's sons eventually relocated from the island of Maui to Oahu with his wife and three daughters, choosing to live at 83 Judd Street, right smack in the midst of some of the most influential early Caucasian immigrants to Hawai'i. These successful missionary families clustered their houses around the property of the first generation of the Judd family, who had also arrived on the *Parthian*.

While many say with tongue in cheek that, "The missionaries came to do good, and they did very well," this family looked after the welfare of my family and, by extension, me. When the Greens of Judd Street saw how many children their cook had, they quickly calculated that my great-grandfather and his brood would not fit in the main house and built a house for him a few blocks away, on Panui Street. The Greens also offered to raise the five eldest girls at their own home. In Hawai'ian culture, new descendants of the royal line were often hidden with trusted friends (*hanai* parents) who adopted them until those children came of age to take up an official position. The Greens were, in a sense, Ah Quan's *hanai* parents.

Their forefather Reverend John had been quite passionate about the importance of educating not just the boys but also Hawai'ian girls, to the extent that he got himself into trouble with the original mission outfitters. Far from having "gone native," I believe Reverend John had made the 148-day journey to Hawai'i with all the best intentions. He had a religious agenda, which included an emphasis on basic education and what would now be considered environmental sustainability practices. He learned to speak the Hawai'ian language (which features as many verb conjugations as Latin) so that he could both teach and preach in the locals' tongue. When he saw the high price of imported wheat, he started a wheat plantation on Maui and taught the locals how to run it. The Green legacy of valuing and sharing education was passed down the Green generations and to me.

The reverend's three granddaughters (Carrie, Rhoda, and Emeline) were at least 30 years older than Ah Quan, but they were very fond of my grandmother and hugely influenced her style and expectations for life. They stayed in touch throughout their lives by letter, and I recognize Ah Quan's voice echoing the upbeat, 1920s flapper-speak of Rhoda's travel missives. Today they would all be bloggers.

Carrie Green was one of the charter librarians at what is now known as the Hawai'i State Library, where I did some of the research for this book. Ah Quan always read and seems never to have been far from a library. In her photo album of pen-pals and school chums at age 15, there are two photos of what is now the Hawai'i State Library. She labeled it, "A Favorite Spot." (What a bookworm she was!) It sits right next door to the royal palace, Iolani, practically kitty-corner to the Mission Houses museum and library, which archived much of the Green family's writings. In her adult married life, Ah Quan continued to be a regular patron of public libraries.

According to 1930 census data, only 25% of American Caucasian women completed a high school education. "Non-whites," as we Asians were categorized at the time, had a graduation rate of less than 9%. Half as many non-white men as women finished high school, likely because they were recruited early to the workforce. Thanks to the tutelage of the missionaries with whom she lived, Ah Quan stood with the graduating class of 1924 at McKinley Public High School. Most of the *haole* (Caucasian) children in Honolulu would have been sent to private schools such as Punahou, instead. In fact, the Green sisters' cousin had been a member of the charter class at Punahou, which is now lauded as President Obama's alma mater.

Sixty years later, the high school graduation rate for my own Asian female cohort is, at 89%, an order of magnitude higher than in Ah Quan's time. I have weighed my potential cognitive reserve against what I know of Ah Quan's, hoping I come out with even greater protective advantages.

Growing up, I enjoyed major "brain success," being always at the top of my class, and while I knew that math was not my strongest subject, it seemed certain that I would get into the university of my choice and follow in the footsteps of my overachieving elder brother, Wingsie, who went to Harvard and then on to chair a department of physics at a ridiculously early age. Of course my parents' friends always asked them what they had done to us, as if they had slipped something into our water or enforced a strict study timetable. A lot of it was just dumb luck: We were lucky in the genes we received from two bright parents. We were lucky to have been born to parents willing to work hard and save to pay tuition for schools where teachers knew how to keep us stimulated. We were lucky to have personalities that make us curious about things, and the pursuit of those interests has earned us the merit badges of scholarship. Things came easily to us until we went to university.

I have had the luxury of never doubting whether I would pursue a university degree—and a choice of profession was wide open to me. My earliest interest in anything medical came from James Herriot's *All Creatures Great and Small*. What young equestrienne didn't get whisked away by that book into a rustic world of devotion to animals? I was inspired by his tireless heroism, his willingness to extend a helping arm up into animals to deliver a newborn unto this earth, and how this contribution was embraced by his community. While I admired Dr. Jim Herriot, I didn't consider myself at all hardy enough to work as a veterinarian or doctor.

When people ask how long it takes to become a neurologist, I'm glad I didn't add it up ahead of time. Of course the first 12 years get you through high school (this doesn't include kindergarten or preschool). During four years of university, I took courses in chemistry, physics, and biology as mandatory preparation for medical school entrance examinations. I was horrified to find my way blocked by chemistry. I had been one of those ninetieth-percentile scorers throughout school, but during my freshman year, I almost failed chemistry. I would have been lucky to get 50% correct on most of the exams! I wonder now if this is what it feels like when our patients are given memory tests in the clinic, and the dementia itself has blotted out insight about how poorly they are performing. It's crushing to think you did something right, only to be told by a dispassionate third party that you didn't even get a passing mark. I try hard not to be that dispassionate third party.

Things eventually improved in my pre-med curriculum. One day, the Head Teaching Assistant for the organic chemistry class tapped me on the shoulder to speak in the hallway outside the auditorium. I thought, "This is it! I'm being escorted out of the building and this university!" My heart was pounding. But that was not the purpose of this meeting. He started out by apologizing for grading errors that had been made by the graduate students scoring my tests. I had not been doing so badly after all! Thank goodness for the concept of partial credit. To this day, I give partial credit on mental status testing for people with English as a second language or hearing impairments or other cultural factors. Perhaps because I struggled so much with my science classes, I was wondering, "Even if Stanford doesn't tire of me, can I get into medical school?" My science grade point average was not competitive. The Head TA couldn't fix my chemistry grades all the way back to year one.

I identified an abrupt disconnect between the excitement I had felt during high school experiences observing an obstetrics/gynecology setting and my struggle through chemistry classes. How could understanding chemistry lead to better skills at interactions with patients? The thing that made me think I had something to offer was the sense that compassion was a key feature for a good physician. And I could do that.

But chemistry persisted as my arch nemesis. I didn't make it into medical school after the first round of applications. So I added a year of master's degree work to my educational tally while I re-applied, this time to some schools that were known for concentrating on clinical skills, as opposed to medical research. In my medical school application essay, I recalled what I had enjoyed at the obstetrics clinic. I tried to stand out by writing that as a physician I would aim to be "The One Who Listened, The One Who Made a Difference." Rush Medical College in Chicago took me in for four years of medical training (for those still counting, we're already at 20 years minimum of education and not licensed yet). For those of you thinking my cognitive reserve had far exceeded that of Ah Quan by this point, sadly the calculation is just not that simple!

My grandparents were proud that I was going to be a doctor and were very supportive of my career pursuit. Ah Quan, of course, knitted me warm things made of acrylics in gaudy colors for the Chicago winters. To be fair, I would have groused if she hadn't adorned me in those, the way she had my brother when he went "up" to Harvard.

I had applied to medical school with no clue about Alzheimer's or amyloid or even that I have a certain talent for working with older patients. I had every intention of specializing in obstetrics and gynecology. I liked the idea of participating in the shiny new beginning of life, not the end of it. I wanted to teach women how to understand their bodies and take better care of themselves. But the hours are rough in that specialty. I don't do well in the wee hours and wouldn't have made as reassuring a coach to first-time mothers as Jamie, the resident showing me the ropes, had been. It is certainly unacceptable to be crankier than the patient in labor. So that specialty was crossed off my list.

Someone convinced me that family medicine could be the match for me. I could still build long-term relationships with patients, I could still work with a focus on preventive medicine, and I would get to know entire families. During the medical school clerkships, which are a sampler of the different special-ties, I learned that family doctors have approximately 11 minutes maximum to spend with each patient, and typically there is just one annual visit. To top it off, the mindset of the well patient is that he doesn't really come to clinic to be told to shed stress-reducing habits, like smoking or substance abuse. Family medicine was therefore out of the running.

The perfect fit of neurology came to me as a surprise. Surgeons like to profess that they can cure disease, saying, "Nothing heals like stainless steel." Before the advent of CT or MRI scanners, neurologists were the antithesis of surgeons in healing efficacy—relatively speaking, if surgeons were wielding lasers in the blinding light of day, neurologists were shooting water guns in the dark. The stereotype was that neurology was an intellectual spectator sport, not really providing services of value to its patients.

The movie *Awakenings* is Oliver Sacks's memoir of trying a medication for Parkinson's disease on patients who had been locked into their inert bodies by complications from a Depression-era flu epidemic. The desired, almost miraculous, effects of the medication wore off by the time the movie's credits rolled, leaving the patients as tragically disabled as they were when the film began. After seeing the movie with my mother, I dreaded the neurology rotation before me: Patients with neurological disorders generally have chronic conditions, and I was anticipating that this rotation would be a real downer. The movie seemed to confirm the reputation of neurology as a series of academic discussions on fascinatingly hopeless cases. But my medical school rotation through neurology (thankfully mandatory for the curriculum) turned this misperception upside down.

One of my first patients with a neurological disorder was an older gentleman who'd had a large left-sided stroke that had suddenly rendered him more than speechless—Howard could not even understand anything that was said to him. All of this had arisen quite suddenly on a Sunday afternoon. In the emergency room, I found his calm in the face of this sudden isolation from language impressive, if not a bit baffling. I can only hope that I would be able to maintain as much poise in the face of such a drastic loss. He was cooperative and seemed to understand that we were trying to help him, but he couldn't answer questions or follow commands and wasn't even able to mimic movements consistently enough to show that he understood what we were saying. Howard had a little right-sided weakness in the face and arm to go with the more severe sign of profound language impairment (neurologists call it *global aphasia*). His condition made me wonder if Howard could still think to himself even though words were not available from within or without. Three days after his stroke, he was still in the hospital for observation and testing.

I was on-call the night he went down to the MRI scanner in the basement for a follow-up brain scan. The first scan had confirmed a large-vessel stroke. The second scan would tell if further complications were impeding his recovery. I happened to be the first to visit with him and his wife upon his return from the scanner in the hospital basement, and I was shocked into muteness myself when he greeted me with, "Well, hello there!" It was as if the Speech Fairy had waved a magic wand. It seemed impossible to me for someone with such a large area of brain affected by stroke to recover so suddenly and after days without improvement.

I was very lucky to witness this. Of course, Howard was even luckier. His wife reported that they'd taken the elevator to the MRI suite, then while they were waiting for their turn, he'd said to her, clearly and in his normal voice, "Haven't I had this done before?" Once I picked my jaw up off the floor, I got cozy on the edge of his bed and asked if he recognized me. He said it felt as if he knew me, I was familiar in a vague way, but he couldn't recall my role as the medical student who had been visiting every morning of his hospital stay.

I asked if he'd been feeling trapped behind a language barrier, wanting to tell us things that wouldn't come out. Howard said, no, that it was more as if he'd just woken up from a heavy, stuporous nap. I was starstruck and proudly presented him to the rest of the team the next morning. He sat up in bed and talked with them as if the whole thing had been just a curious dream.

That case made the specialty-choice decision for me: I was to become a neurologist. Here was a man who had suddenly met criteria for dementia (unable to communicate, unable to show decision making or memory function secondary to the aphasia) and then, just as suddenly, had gotten *himself* out of it, without use of any of the interventions we now have for acute stroke reversal. Howard raised all sorts of philosophical questions in my mind about how important retaining language ability is to someone's thought processes: What kind of quality of life can one have after being rendered aphasic? What kind of memory function do you have if you don't have words? Was it important for Howard not to have been aware of his condition in order to spare him the anxiety it caused in others? How much of a person's cognition can you whittle away and still have the same person before you? Is the soul in the brain? I also had to wonder about what role, if any, medical care had played in Howard's recovery.

Neurology was the right fit for me. When someone has a neurological problem, he is motivated to have a dialogue with the physician: "How did this happen? How can I make it go away? What will happen over time?" Patients and their families ask questions, do reading on their own, and build a relationship with me and the staff that lasts years.

After settling on this career path, there was one year of internship, and three years of neurology residency training. After 24 years, I could hang my shingle as a neurologist. While in residency training, I realized that I have a really soft spot in my heart for older patients. I attribute part of that to the cultural respect my parents taught me for our elders.

It was during my residency that Ah Quan died. Ah Quan's stroke proved an index event for me as a physician. My parents, although always supportive of pursuing education, had had mixed feelings about my application to medical school. Friends of theirs in medicine were not happy with the advent of health maintenance organizations (HMOs) and the relative loss of medical decision making and billing autonomy for doctors in the United States. My parents were much more taken by the idea of my continuing to study marine biology and becoming the next Jacques Cousteau.

But on the day that I walked into Ah Quan's hospital room with my mother, introduced myself to my grandmother's geriatrician, reviewed her vital signs with the nurses, and held her CT scans up to the fluorescent ceiling lights to review, my mother realized that I *was* a doctor, not a documentarist for *National Geographic*.

For her, it all came together in those few moments. In her words, "You just walked in there wearing a pair of blue jeans, but there they were, treating you like a doctor!" I had finished medical school and completed most of my residency already, with staff at three hospitals addressing me as "Doctor," but there's nothing like having a parent come to that first recognition that I have grown up, bear a title, and most importantly, am in a position to help other people in a significant way.

To subspecialize in dementia took another three years of training, called a fellowship. Most academic clinicians do a two- to three-year fellowship after residency, and this brings the total of my years of formal education to 27. I continue to learn daily, of course—from my colleagues and my patients. All of which, I hope, will build up my cognitive reserve.

How does the cognitive reserve shield our brains? The Nun Study by David Snowdon's group reports that higher educational levels will help the brain to develop additional ways of thinking and problem solving that render it more resistant to Alzheimer's disease. One measure in the Nun Study was a review of essays that the novitiates had written on entry to the convent. These essays would not have been influenced by duration of residence or training received at the convent, and they were taken as proxies of the educational level and perhaps intelligence of the young women. As a validation of this choice, researchers also studied writing samples of the same individuals at later intervals over the rest of their lives and found that writing styles did not tend to change throughout their adult lives.

In specific, idea density and grammatical structure were scored in these writing samples. Someone with a sixth-grade-level achievement or lower might write something fairly straightforward in her autobiography, such as, "I was born in Los Angeles, California." A novitiate with a higher level of education and some writing experience might have incorporated more ideas: "They say it never rains in California, but I was born in the middle of a dark and stormy night in the City of Angels, 3000 miles away from this convent."

The nuns from this order very generously consented in advance to brain autopsy so that the researchers could look for differences in Alzheimer's pathology between nuns eventually diagnosed with Alzheimer's disease and those who died of other causes. Those nuns with the higher idea density and grammatical structure scores fared well during life despite the presence of Alzheimer's disease plaques and tangles in their brains.

In a second report from this study sample, evidence from the nuns showed two things: Not only did education help to stave off development of Alzheimer's disease but also, where two brain problems are present, there is a cumulative effect on cognition. Specifically, cerebrovascular disease or strokes plus Alzheimer's pathology almost guarantees that the person will show outward signs of impairment, such as progressive worsening of memory loss, whereas other sisters with Alzheimer's pathology and no other neurological illness was much less likely to exhibit significant memory loss before she died. It is not yet clear whether a person has only the first two decades of life to build such cognitive reserve.

Ah Quan loved to write. I was able to locate columns she had written during her career at the Hawai'i Board of Water Supply, to score her pieces for idea density and grammatical structure. Her column was called *Ka Waipuna*, which means "Spring from the Resources" in English:

> *July 1958*
>
> *Water Resources is being renovated and some day, real soon we hope, we can settle down. This is a time of utter confusion and it's just good luck and/or an elephant's memory—or both, that we can find things. Please shut your eyes as you walk by! Is there a brave soul in this building who hasn't instinctively shuddered when that giant drill went c-a-r-a-n-g? For him a royal purple heart! When the whistle blows at 4:30 P.M. we troop out, feeling as though every single tooth in our heads has taken an all-out drilling. All this and the heat too—no wonder we're all shook up. Oh well, it can't last forever, thank goodness. Come and see us when we're all prettied up.*

For idea density (the average number of ideas expressed per 10 words within a block of 10 sentences), Ah Quan scores 7.5, which was about the same as the average nun per Snowdon's methods, despite the wit in her words. For grammatical complexity, she scored at most 5.0 out of 7.0 on one of the sentences, but was otherwise a bit below the average nun. Any advantage of idea density appears to have been balanced back to neutral by the grammatical complexity score, so if Ah Quan had been a participant in the Nun Study, the investigators would have placed her among those who would be no better at staving off Alzheimer's disease than anyone else.

I think that, despite her relatively low scores, Ah Quan's cognitive reserve did help her. As Ah Quan lived past her eightieth year, we noted that she was making some mistakes, but there was no overt evidence of dementia. Like many others of her generation, experience had taught her to be frugal, and she would let no food go to waste. Plastic bags of food in the refrigerator were labeled as to contents and date of storage. In her later years, Ah Quan was putting plastic bags containing disposed bones or gristle into the refrigerator alongside the juicy slices of Pirie mango from their yard.

She continued typewriting her correspondence to family and friends in those years. She was so good at touch-typing that she had stopped looking at the keyboard decades prior. It was not unusual for the entire letter to arrive in unintentional code, letters shifted over to the right or left by one line of keys. We recipients across the Pacific were more entertained than alarmed by the secret code. It was a message to be exchanged among our League of Typists, especially since translation of those letters revealed that Ah Quan remembered vividly everyone's genealogies, recipes, grandchildren's birthdays, and recent sales on lamb chops at the local grocery store (where she frequently ran into Jack Lord of the original *Hawaii Five-O* series).

We attributed Ah Quan's minor mistakes to her visual loss, not Alzheimer's disease. She had macular degeneration, and that provided sufficient explanation. I theorize that Ah Quan's academic successes and vibrant community involvement (see Chapter 10, Social Networks) helped offset the Alzheimer's pathology that she must have been harboring at the time. The deposition of amyloid in her arteries to cause that fatal bleeding had not occurred overnight.

By the time most people hear about this positive effect of education, it is already too late. They have finished their formal schooling, or the circumstances of their upbringing did not allow them to determine for themselves how much education they would pursue. This raises all sorts of interesting questions, such as, "What is it about higher educational level that is so protective?" The flip side of the question is, of course, whether whatever enables pursuit of higher education—intrinsic brain power or environmental circumstances such as socioeconomic status—protects you, as opposed to the schooling itself. Which came first, the chicken or the egg?

One study has shown that a high literacy level (something that you can increase later in life), can slow the onset of dementia among those who are otherwise at high genetic risk.

What evidence do we have that IQ or intelligence level plays a role in cognitive reserve? Everyone agrees that both genetic and environmental factors determine your intelligence. Author Malcolm Gladwell has written about the phenomenon of the person with the highest-percentile IQ not succeeding in life, based on environmental circumstances that did not offer opportunities to capitalize on his strengths.

Gladwell argues that the individual in today's North American society requires more than what we call "book smarts": She needs to wield a certain "EQ" (for "emotional quotient"), which was previously known as "people skills." In the same way, different types of intelligence may interact to set up an individual as someone who is likely to develop many shortcuts or back routes for managing brain processes. When a person develops coronary artery disease slowly, the arteries create extra branches and ways to get around cholesterol plugs to deliver blood to the heart muscle itself. Those extra arterial connections are called *collaterals*. The combination of several cognitive strengths likely sets up collaterals against injuries to the brain. I believe it is the collateral system encouraged by cognitive reserve that bolsters resilience against Alzheimer's changes, not specifically high test scores.

There are eight types of intelligence, not just school smarts and emotional intelligence, and those eight do overlap in function and expression. One type is "high verbal acumen" (or "good with words"), which generally forms the basis for IQ scores. Your intelligence quotient score includes both a verbal score and a performance score. Your school career may have been made or broken by your first IQ testing session: Children who do well on admission tests are slated for smaller class sizes and an enriched curriculum, which offers additional advantages for academic success. Generally, people gifted in logic and reasoning intelligence make good candidates for law school. A visuospatial intelligence facilitates remembering where things are in space and being able to manipulate images or objects in your head, keeping track of the object's left and right sides, no matter what the orientation. There is a similar type of intelligence that we would attribute to athletes, in that they are very adept at orienting bodies in space. There is a musical intelligence, which many of us believe has to do with the same type of strength as language but uses the non-language hemisphere of the brain. Interpersonal intelligence is the "EQ" popularized recently. People with *intra*personal intelligence are in closer touch with their own feelings, motivations, and goals; they may be more introverted as a result. The eighth type of intelligence concerns the natural world, and that refers to the physics of things; for example, knowing how far from the edge of the railing a dropped egg may land without giving it a trial shove first.

It may be better for overall lifetime success to have talents at a moderate level in two or more of these areas, as opposed to being a superstar in one and having no aptitude in the rest. When we test individuals to monitor whether cognition has declined, we use their careers and hobbies to anticipate where their strengths and weaknesses may lie. For example, the stereotypical mechanical engineer should perform in the high average range (or better) on tests from the visuospatial and mathematical calculation domains, since we are expecting him or her to have visuospatial and natural world intelligence. The practical applications of mechanical engineering might also raise logic and reasoning scores.

If that patient registers borderline impaired scores on those tasks and the complaint is, "I think I'm losing it, but no one else seems to notice," we often find that the person is still functioning independently and therefore doesn't meet criteria for dementia, but our index of suspicion goes up. Perhaps this mechanical engineer is in the early stage of Alzheimer's disease or another dementia. Variables that increase the likelihood of Alzheimer's would include the patient's age, a history of Alzheimer's disease in a parent or sibling, and an observation that short-term memory is failing ("I can't remember where we went out for dinner last night," *as opposed to*, "I can't remember who the sixteenth U.S. president was").

Alternatively, high blood pressure, diabetes, and smoking in the same patient might make us look for a stroke as the cause of these relative cognitive deficits. If, on neurological examination, the patient had some stiffness of the muscles on passive movement and slowing of initiation of movement, we might suspect that the patient has an early stage of Parkinson's disease. Or if, on speaking with someone who knows the patient well, we find that these subtle cognitive changes are actually accompanied by some major character changes, the diagnosis of frontotemporal dementia would be considered.

Cognitive reserve and educational level are important to consider in the evaluation of a patient with cognitive impairment, and the evidence points to some protective effects of higher education. But there are many other contributors to dementia risk and the depth to which cognition will be impaired.

4

PLASTICITY

Is the brain like a muscle? Does one use it or lose it? Scientists have learned that higher educational levels allow us to build up cognitive reserve, akin to the concept of saving money in the bank for an unforeseen crisis. But in order to keep the brain supple, it's important to keep learning new activities or skills throughout life.

When a brain is forced to make new connections to perform a new skill, plasticity is maintained. Plasticity refers to the idea that the brain can recover, redeem itself, or simply continue to grow connections over a lifetime. This relatively new discovery has brought hope to the practice of neurology. We marine biologists know that a starfish can regenerate a severed arm, but the brain is more complex. It needs to start with new neuronal sprouts, then continue through accurate growth trails from those budding neurons along intricately nested circuits.

A fully developed brain is connected so that each piece of information is cross-referenced many times over (we don't even know how many!). With maximized interconnectivity, one associative link between events can give high-speed access to insights or problem solving. Dementia reverses this process, subtracting connections due to relentless neurodegenerative disorders. For patients with dementia, triggering plasticity is a means of countering that erasure.

In residency, I read with interest of bold experiments that implanted early fetal tissue in Parkinson's disease patients. While this practice led to an increase in tissue in the desired location, the new sprouts didn't know where to connect; ultimately, the experiment failed to improve patients' control over their movements. Imagine the starfish with four normal-sized arms and one tiny-sized armlet, then a month later with five normal-sized arms but the new one drags behind the rest of the animal. This is not helpful, and actually endangers the animal by slowing it down for predators.

One form of plasticity works by guiding neuronal sprouts into destinations where they can settle into harmony within a working network. That is still very much a work in progress. We have some clues: A chemical known as brain-derived neurotrophic factor gives brain cells the "Go" signal to sprout and extend. Physical exercise can increase the brain's release of this chemical, but we have yet to figure out how to use any cognitive exercise to reverse memory loss.

Another form of brain plasticity is the re-appropriation of existing brain regions into new function, which is a bit like getting neurons to switch hats. A stunning example of this has been described by Dr. Pawan Sinha, professor of computational neuroscience at the Massachusetts Institute of Technology, who has brought sight to Southeast Asian children who have waited too long for congenital cataract treatment. These children were born with a reversible blindness. In North America, most children are treated immediately after the diagnosis has been made, but Dr. Sinha recognized that in India most of these potential surgical patients were left blind, which markedly endangers their lives and stunts their development.

Some of the children who have had their cataracts removed through his program had already grown into their late teens. Would the surgery work on brain regions that had been lying fallow, without visual input? In a nutshell, yes. And immediately! What their brains perceived at first as a splatter of stimuli was processed later as object patterns that could be more quickly recognized whole. Consider a circle overlapping with a square. To a visual rookie, the lines would look like a tangle, not two objects superimposed. With some computer-facilitated training, Dr. Sinha's newly sighted patients were able to quickly identify a circle and hexagon from within a jumble of lines. They then needed a few months to catch up on learning to read and other visually based skills, but they could do it! Once the eyes can register light, it takes only days for the patients' brains, even after two decades of blindness, to process that brand-new sensory mode. Dr. Sinha's work is inspirational not only because of its humanitarian scope but also because of the knowledge it has yielded about brain plasticity.

In the past decade, we have heard the good news that the adult brain can develop or reinforce connections between cells. Neurorehabilitation now emphasizes re-establishing broken lines of communication in the brain. Although plasticity is most apparent in parts of the brain that manage movement, it is taking longer to find the right interventions to reconnect lost cognitive functions. Applying ideas about plasticity to help return the brain to a higher level of function has not yet worked well for cases of dementia. Trying to fix something after the problem has already occurred has been likened to shutting the barn door after the horse that was inside has already bolted. Is the horse already out of the barn once a patient is diagnosed with dementia?

Those families who have had the sudden gift of a "normal" or insightful conversation with a patient, after years of decline, wonder, "Where did that come from? Has he been able but just not connected all this time? What put him back online and then switched him off to inaccessible so abruptly?" The answers to those questions are unclear, but the immediate reaction whenever such a brief awakening occurs is to figure out how to make it happen again. Was there a change in sleep pattern, diet, or physical health that brought this on? My informal observation is that this tends to occur within two months before the patient's death, which defies my current understanding of neurodegeneration and raises the unscientific but natural hope that the patient is somehow being granted a last chance to communicate. An event like this raises hope that it would be possible to jump-start those brain connections, no matter the length of illness. Likewise, the ideal cognitive rehabilitation would allow patients to benefit from stimulation of the brain at any age, whether that was to redevelop connections that help them move their arms in a more coordinated way after a stroke, or to reconnect those networks that have been targeted by dementing illness.

We haven't gained much ground in restoring mental faculties, but a large new business is booming in preventative cognitive rehab, which is more like training the brain to run well through the marathon of life's challenges. The lay public has no doubt heard that playing video games or solving sudoku puzzles or playing mahjong in mid-life can help prevent Alzheimer's disease. There are occasionally articles that show the benefits of such activity, but it's hard to do a study that would apply to every person. Our intellectual strengths and weaknesses require different activities for maintenance and for enhancement. You may even be wondering whether those who are past formal schooling can cheat Alzheimer's by doing mental exercises that pump up cognitive reserve. This is the current billion-dollar question.

Video game developers are in hot competition to create something that shows results. Early experiments indicate that the video games teach one how to play each game well in turn. These games' positive effects on real-life functions—like remembering what to pick up at the grocery store or how to prepare a six-course meal for company—have not been shown convincingly yet, but creating something that will extrapolate to real-life improvements may be a matter of improving game design. The downside of spending more time in front of a computer is that it takes away from time for social networking, which is also important for maintaining the brain's plasticity.

What about sitting in front of a television screen? One research group has found an added 33% risk of late-life cognitive impairment among those who report daily TV watching during mid-life. The problem may not be the television itself, but rather because other sedentary habits that are highly associated with television viewing are also linked to obesity and physically unsuccessful aging, which are themselves risk factors for dementia.

Friends and relatives send me newspaper clippings claiming that playing mahjong can prevent the onset of dementia. But one wonders whether there is an association between the game and preserved cognitive function that isn't quite causal. I have yet to see someone explore whether other aspects of life that enable regular mahjong playing—such as being healthy enough to be independently mobile and able to interact successfully in social situations—are more responsible for the benefit than the mahjong itself. Or maybe it's the practice of one of the card-playing skills (the scoring math or the tracking of how many cards of the desired suit have been called onto the board during the game) that is more important than the specific game played.

One study specifically trained participants to hone memory ("What were the 10 words I just read out loud to you?"), reasoning ("If Neil is taller than William and William is taller than John, is John shorter than Neil?"), or processing speed ("Connect the dots as quickly and accurately as you can"). When participating in any cognitive training program, subjects were able to improve their scores in that one cognitive domain over a five-year period. The initial training alone was fairly significant as an intervention. Booster sessions over the five-year period seemed to help a bit. But it's important to note that better memory did not translate to improvements in the untrained areas of reasoning or processing speed. This reinforces to me that if you want to maintain a variety of cognitive activities, perfecting one cognitive parlor trick is not enough to protect you over time.

One study maintained that people older than 65 can benefit from several cognitively stimulating activities like doing crosswords, playing cards, attending organizations, or going to the cinema or theater; if sustained regularly, these activities seem to delay the onset of dementia. In contrast, activities that are deemed passive (watching television, listening to the radio, listening to music, knitting, and sewing) were found to be less effective at preventing the onset of dementia. I was perturbed to see that the authors of this paper had designated knitting and sewing as passive activity. None of them could ever have started a pattern for a cable-knit sweater! My grandmother is tsk-tsking from among the macadamia nut trees where her ashes were spread. However, activities they deemed to be cognitively stimulating were more protective than physical activities (such as exercise and odd jobs).

Other researchers regard leisure activity as something that maintains, not enhances, brain function. Continuing one's prior routines would maintain brain function; attending lectures on new topics or learning a new board game or dance would enhance brain function. If the intent is to restructure how to spend leisure time as a result of reading this, consider participating in routine activities more frequently, as that regularity can be as important to maintaining brain function as new activities are to enhancing it.

Despite differences in their design, studies consistently endorse certain strategies as effective for brain health: engagement in the world, maintaining past routines, and making a regular effort to try something new. It's also noteworthy that a lifelong reading habit is a better predictor of how slowly Alzheimer's disease may progress than is IQ or educational level. Reading—while considered a passive activity by the previously mentioned researchers—can challenge the brain to retain new facts or develop different points of view. Those who have not been steady readers in the past can still benefit from adopting a reading habit later in life. Some research groups have suggested that late-life leisure activities may grant protective effects similar to the benefits bestowed by a higher educational level.

Ah Quan would chuckle to know that reading is so important. She was a public library user throughout her life, thanks to the missionaries. My grandmother and I connected over books. Years after she had introduced me to the book, I re-read *That Quail, Robert* when I inherited Ah Quan's copy and gained an entirely different appreciation for the story. As a child, I'd enjoyed the idea of a wild bird becoming a pet, but as an adult, I realized that the charm of the tale is in the loving telling. The author, Robert's human "mom," describes everything about this bird—both the good and the less flattering—with wonder, appreciation, delight, and full acceptance. She and her husband and their friends were devoted to this phenomenal encounter with nature and enjoyed it to the fullest. She also had the talent to sketch the quail in ways that captured its most endearing features. What a great example she gives of engaging her brain in her various passions.

The concept of brain plasticity takes many forms, but to me, the macro view of plasticity is reflected in how one addresses changes in life. This can be especially meaningful to caregivers and how they learn to expect and manage change. From what I have read and learned from my patients, I have come to value the perspective that all things will change. The goal should be to adapt to those changes either as a couple or as a community, instead of struggling to control everything out of craving or aversion. This is a psychological kind of plasticity.

Practicing equanimity, compassion, and loving kindness during changes impacts how the brain reacts to the adversity of change. Brain regions that handle emotional swings and the release of anxiety-causing chemicals can be trained to respond with less hypersensitivity. Equanimity keeps us mindful of the impermanence of things, no matter how comfortable we may find them. It teaches us that there is peace to be gained by avoiding rigid emotional attachments to any one circumstance.

Given that we are all interconnected and that it is the nature of things to change, the path to a peaceful existence includes embracing the impermanence of life events. One of the truths that I've learned, respected, and appreciated is that regardless of the diagnosis and correct identification of the abnormal protein perpetrator, dementia is about change. Humans are exquisitely wired to adapt to change, even if those transformations are not what we wanted or expected. In the stories I've included in this book, I have seen surprising and inspirational capacities for change, not only in the affected patients, but also in their family members and friends. When a patient begins to show signs of dementia, whether behavioral disturbance or memory loss, his life is changing. But so are the lives of everyone close to him. Not all of these changes are for the worse, but it is challenging to have to make these adjustments, and the dementia is usually unexpected.

An acquaintance became one of my most important teachers about change. Bill called me shortly after I moved to Toronto to see if I was attending the twenty-fifth wedding anniversary of mutual friends in Los Angeles. He also mentioned that he had developed some problems with words, which was a big concern for him as a lawyer. Yet he didn't seem to be having any difficulty with word-finding while we were on the phone, and I knew that he had been pushing himself very hard, working long hours, exercising less than usual, and maxing out on stress. When I met him, Bill tended to be self-centered, and I imagined that his new cognitive complaint was a means of trying to glean some extra attention from me. I saw him at the party the following month and he seemed fine, but then six weeks later I received a call from a friend of his: Bill had experienced an excruciating headache and then lost consciousness, and now the staff at the emergency room were saying that he had had a stroke. Working against that snap diagnosis was the fact that Bill had been the quintessential health nut, with no body fat, extreme vegetarian habits, and huge bottles of vitamin supplements that rattled in his carry-on bags back and forth across the United States wherever he tried cases. He seemed like the last person on earth who would have a stroke. I dreaded something worse.

Indeed, a few hours later I got another phone call, this time informing me that Bill had a brain tumor. Given his age of 45 and the tumor's location, I not only had an explanation for his word-finding difficulty, but also knew that his days on the planet were numbered. I finally got to talk to him on the phone the next day, prior to the surgery to remove a part of the tumor to confirm the diagnosis. There had been a major psychological transformation.

In the 24 hours since receiving his diagnosis, he had gained an entirely new perspective on life. It wasn't quite like the Grinch Who Stole Christmas finding his heart growing three sizes, but Bill had suddenly accepted that he did not have control over life, and that searching for perfection might blind him to the kindness and beauty surrounding him. He was able to reach this realization so quickly because he had been studying meditation and Buddhism his entire adult life.

Bill's spirituality was news to me. In our few prior inter-actions, I had been subjected to long monologues about expensive red wine, name-dropping about famous thinkers or writers, and treatises on the intricacies of scuba diving. Bill's complete turnaround was cause for joy and celebration. He said himself that if he had to choose between having a brain tumor and remaining the obnoxious playboy lawyer he'd been, he would take the tumor. We often give brain tumor patients high-dose steroids to reduce the swelling around the tumor, and there may be some hypomania or giddiness associated with steroid use at this level. Over time, however, Bill proved that his new and improved attitude was not just a steroid high.

Everyone's initial reason for coming to my clinic is to reverse the initial stages of cognitive impairment or to prevent the advancement of the underlying illness. In the case of Alzheimer's disease and the other most common causes of dementia, there is nothing to reverse or halt the progression of the illness, which forces us to focus on other issues that contribute to the quality of life for the patient and for those closest to her. Each family member or close friend has a different timetable for making the transition from fighting the disease to accepting that life has changed and will continue to change, in ways that cannot be anticipated. I view that shift from railing against a mystery disease to managing an irreversible dementia as a "Dance of Negotiation."

In order for the health care team to work with the patient and family, we all have to be able to move together to achieve our common goals. It is easy for us to start by agreeing that we all want the patient to feel well. But the health care team has to regulate how it imparts information to correspond with each family's ability to hear, understand, and implement the diagnosis and appropriate management plan. It is a dance, because the patient cannot benefit until we are all moving together, through a mutual understanding of roles, decision making, and leadership.

I flew down to Florida several times to visit Bill in the last 18 months of his life. There I learned that he had shelves of books by Thich Nhat Hanh, the Dalai Lama, and other teachers of dharma and meditation. Contrary to most expectations, it was much less distressing to be with him, even as his body dwindled from the tumor, than to let the mind wander to a future time when he would no longer be with us. He took time to reconcile relationships and to make sure that people knew he cared about them. He apologized for having previously excluded small children and animals from his home. He reveled in the loving support he received from his family and friends.

There were also instances when he sadly and exhaustedly acknowledged how sick the medication was making him feel. I valued his new, refreshing honesty in our interactions. It had an enriched range—from the humor of his warning to expect Jabba the Hutt to meet me at the airport (with Jabba being how he thought of his new, steroid-induced appearance) to the sadness of knowing his mother would have to survive his passing. Gone were the name-dropping monologues. He asked me to tell him what was going on with his brain and his medication and what choices he had about continuing or stopping his care. He spoke about having to put on a brave face for some visitors, and wishing that he had more downtime to continue his meditation practice but knowing that he had to balance his daily schedule to accommodate visiting well-wishers. When we talked, we could be open about the fact that he likely would not be around in the following year. Bill turned out to be quite adept at the Dance of Negotiation.

The steps of that Dance resemble Elisabeth Kübler-Ross's five stages of grief: denial, anger, bargaining, depression, and acceptance. It can take a long time to admit that symptoms of dementia are occurring, generally out of fear of what that means for the future. This can be followed by dissatisfaction or confusion regarding the information available about dementia, about how to get the patient evaluated properly, then about how the doctor has arrived at the diagnosis of dementia. People might wonder, "Why isn't there more to be done? Are the tests accurate? Why don't all the tests have to declare the same conclusion in order for the doctor to feel certain about the diagnosis? If I go to another doctor and he says something different, whom should I believe?" It's hard for patients and their loved ones to feel any peace of mind amid all those concerns.

Going through Bill's terminal illness with him showed me how important it is to facilitate the acceptance phase. The health care team needs to diminish fears in order that the patient and family can adapt to their markedly changed circumstances.

Once I'd learned from Bill how he viewed his tumor and prognosis—with honesty, bravery, and compassion for himself— we could enjoy being in the same emotional space, with similar expectations, hopes, and regrets. We could joke: He wanted me to read Yann Martel's *Life of Pi*, and I agreed, only "to honor a dying man's wish." He knew that most people's first reaction to seeing him was, "Boy, am I glad it's you and not me," and he could tease them about it. Once, during his final weeks, he woke up in the hospice to find me and another friend, Tom Neuman, camped out at the foot of his bed, and said, "Geez, it looks like you guys are sittin' there waiting for me to die!" I recall Tom's response (he's the one who teaches that the patient is always having a worse day than the doctor) as, "Well, duh! We are!" followed by laughter and tears. We can upset ourselves mourning in advance for someone with a terminal illness, or we can sit with him and say, "I am really going to be sad when you are gone, but what can I do for you today, while we're both sitting here together?" In the last 18 months of his life, Bill used to call me out of the blue, just because he was grateful for the fact that he still could. Those calls were occasions for joy, and as with the other three Buddhist practices, our joy did not arise from turning away from pain and suffering. Instead, joy flourishes within practicing compassion for those who are suffering, extending loving kindness, and keeping oneself open to the possibilities that change offers.

As a marine biologist and now neurologist, I appreciate that every living thing with a nervous system shies away from painful or noxious situations and that we are electrically wired to feel some sense of reward when something pleasurable is happening. One primary urge in life is to avoid suffering. The trick is not to get caught up in a reactionary stance that reduces existence to a series of reflexive acts, much like the behavior of a barnacle. If avoiding suffering is the only goal, life becomes a matter of clinging to comfortable situations and hiding from uncomfortable ones. When it comes to dealing with dementia, the exact opposite is demanded.

5

DID I INHERIT ALZHEIMER'S FROM AH QUAN?

My grandmother and I are both Fire Horses. According to Chinese astrology, Fire Horse women are headstrong and their uncontrollably independent nature presents an element of danger. The Fire Horse enjoys spectacular luck, whether good or terribly tragic; for us, there is nothing in moderation. This description runs akin to the Western zodiac sign of Aquarius, "destined for madness or greatness." On the positive side, Horses are regarded as outgoing, people-loving, ambitious and popular leaders, noble, strong, and freedom-loving. The addition of the Fire modifier to a Chinese Horse brings on traits of impulsiveness and inability to take feedback well. But these are exactly the characteristics that can benefit medical researchers. We have to be willing to take risks for innovative ideas and compete for shrinking support from funding agencies; as well, we have to sell the idea of research participation to interested patients and their families. Regardless of whether one follows astrological charts, most people do believe that genetics can influence our lives.

Three generations—Ah Quan, my mother, and I—bear an uncanny facial resemblance. We all share a distinct preference for sweets, we all enjoy written correspondence with friends from all over the globe (Ah Quan would have loved email), and our voices are so alike that when Ah Quan spent the holidays at our house in Los Angeles, her callers couldn't tell which of the three of us had answered the phone. The evidence that I bear a large share of Ah Quan's DNA seems incontestable. For the most part, these are points of pride, but I do want to avoid Ah Quan's Alzheimer's disease.

Arguably, Ah Quan benefited from a quick end to her life and not the long, difficult descent into dementia that most people associate with Alzheimer's disease. Ah Quan did not seem to have any of the typical features of Alzheimer's disease. She was never "failing," but it is also hard to know how much Grandpa was helping her to compensate for any problems. My grandparents' daily routine started with gardening early in the morning to beat the hot Hawai'ian sun, followed by trips to the supermarket, library, and post office, by social visits, and by letter writing. They did everything together in their retirement years, and if my grandfather had taken on a more supervisory role over time, it might have happened so gradually and required so little time and energy overall that even he was not aware of it.

Richard Bach points out in *Illusions* that often the people who turn out to be family don't all share the same blood; family can be chosen. But biological parents are not chosen by their children, and there's no altering the genetic makeup parents passed on to their children. There are some genetic mutations associated with familial Alzheimer's disease, but they account for fewer than 10% of Alzheimer's cases.

Many readers will have learned about Mendelian genetics in high school. This is enough to understand that the body is mostly using parental genes as a blueprint for how it will appear and function. In the Mendelian explanation of genetics, there are some versions of genes that dominate others and some gene versions that work together to create a blended appearance or function.

Do you remember the pea flowers that Gregor Mendel described? Pollen from a red flower used to fertilize the female part of another red flower would result in seeds that grew into plants with red flowers. The same holds true for white flower "parents." But combining a red parent plant and a white parent plant results in a red offspring, when the red gene is dominant over the white. If the red and the white genes did not respect a dominance hierarchy, a pink flower would result.

If the genetics of Alzheimer's disease worked according to this simple format, it might be much easier to predict one's own risk of getting Alzheimer's disease once a parent was diagnosed. The statistics would work something like this: If the father's Alzheimer's disease were caused by a gene that was transmitted regardless of the sex of the child, each child would have a fifty-fifty chance of getting Alzheimer's disease. (*Sex*, by the way, refers to the XX or XY chromosomal determination of an individual; *gender* denotes how the individual identifies him- or herself to more typically masculine or feminine roles within the culture.) Conversely, if the Alzheimer's disease in one parent were due to a recessive gene, the child would develop Alzheimer's disease only if that child were to inherit a second recessive Alzheimer's gene from the other parent. However, genetic explanations for why patients have developed

Alzheimer's disease have remained exceedingly difficult to identify.

Patients' family members ask me about genetic risk all the time. One heart-rending scenario in my clinic featured a patient in her fifties with progressive memory loss who nursed her mother through a terrible course of illness with Alzheimer's disease, only to recognize the same symptoms in herself a short time later. Only two years after her mother died, Petra herself began to note short-term memory loss and problems finding words. She turned to her husband and children at the clinic visit where we confirmed her diagnosis of Alzheimer's disease and comforted *them*, reassuring them that it would be all right and that God had intended it to be this way. What a bold woman.

As her illness progressed, she became paranoid about her family and her home. Every time we counseled her husband, he cried openly about the loss of their future (they had not even retired before her illness set in). He experienced so much stress in trying to care for her himself—out of grief and out of guilt, and to the exclusion of their adult children—that he suffered a stress-induced heart attack. After that point, he did accept the help of his children and other community resources.

Fortunately, this is not a common scenario in Alzheimer's. Only a very small percentage of people in the world carry an indelible familial pattern of inheritance of Alzheimer's. Nevertheless, the statistics for the last 15 years have shown that if a parent or another first-degree relative such as a sibling or a child has Alzheimer's disease, a person's risk of developing Alzheimer's disease triples. It is not yet clear how to translate that through two generations—what is the impact if a grandparent but not a parent was affected? That's where the Mendelian explanation of genetics falls short. Over time, we have come to understand that the many factors within a person's environment (such as multiple head traumas or educational level) interact with his or her genetic makeup to eventually allow or deny dementia a foothold.

Add a degree of complexity: The *ways* in which people interact with their environment may also be determined by their genetic structure. For example, some people are more prone to depression when they are under stressful conditions than others are, based on their genetics. And major depressive disorder is a risk factor for Alzheimer's disease. Some people are genetically inclined to seek extreme adventure, which indirectly raises the risk for head trauma, which is itself a risk factor for cognitive impairment.

Modern-day courses in genetics now breeze very quickly past the simple principles of Mendelian genetics to a more advanced understanding of the nuances of one's genetic makeup, or genotype, that can contribute to risks for Alzheimer's disease. The next level of sophistication in genetics focuses on subsections of the gene. These are such short sequences of information that they are also referred to by a short name: SNPs (pronounced "snips"). *SNP* stands for *single nucleotide polymorphism*. Two individuals' genetic codes for a particular protein may differ by only one very small SNP element. This means that you and I can have genes that differ by one element (we have two different SNPs), without making significantly different protein products. Often, several versions of a SNP lead to a genetic product constructed in the same amount with the same range of function. Other SNPs may lead to an advantage in either the level of production of the protein in the body or the way in which that protein functions. Still other SNPs may lead to an outright disadvantage.

The most frequently mentioned SNP in relation to Alzheimer's disease is the set of variations on Apolipoprotein E. Apolipoprotein E is a protein that sets us and chimpanzees apart from the rest of the primates, and its function is to help us manage cholesterol gleaned from meat eating. Although not many genetic culprits for Alzheimer's disease have been identified (recall my "10% of cases" figure above), Apolipoprotein E remains the genetic finding most frequently related to risk of Alzheimer's disease, and of course I wonder if my mother, brother, or I have the "wrong" type.

In the 1990s, the description of Apolipoprotein E and its relationship to Alzheimer's disease caused many patients and their physicians to order genetic testing to see if individuals with family histories, and even those without, had the type of Apolipoprotein E that contributes to Alzheimer's disease. If this gene were to work like a Mendelian dominance hierarchy, testing might have been useful, but Apolipoprotein E does not follow the Mendelian inheritance pattern.

Pairs of SNPs determine the versions of Apolipoprotein E numbered ε2, ε3, or ε4. Each version contributes differently to a person's risk of developing Alzheimer's disease. Whether one has ε2, ε3, or ε4 depends on the pair of SNPs present in genes for Apolipoprotein E. This is an example of how it may take more than one SNP variation to change an outcome. Each of us carries two copies of the gene, which means that a person may have two copies of ε2 or a combination of two types, such as ε2 + ε3 or ε2 + ε4, and so on.

I realize this starts to sound like the red and white flowers sometimes making a pink flower, but don't go there! It is different. In general, people harboring one copy of ε4 are at a higher risk for Alzheimer's disease than people without any copies of ε4; a person who has two copies of ε4 (we call this person a *homozygote*) is at even higher risk of developing Alzheimer's disease. But 25% of the population has one or more ε4! Studies vary in approximating the risk of Alzheimer's disease in those with the double dose of ε4: By age 85, the homozygote may have between 50% and 90% risk of having Alzheimer's disease. The homozygote with Alzheimer's disease in a first-degree relative will have a risk level right up at 90%. That can sound pretty ominous, but the three most important points to keep in mind are: (1) ε2 is apparently protective against getting Alzheimer's disease; (2) the presence of one or two ε4 copies is not sufficient to produce Alzheimer's disease; and (3) the presence of one or two ε4 copies is not *necessary* to produce Alzheimer's disease. ε2 has its dark side: Carriers of ε2 tend to have more problems managing their cholesterol and therefore may have higher risk of stroke or heart attack, instead of Alzheimer's disease.

A carrier is a person whose genes have been tested but who is not manifesting the illness of interest. I had mixed feelings reading recently that Apolipoprotein ε4 carriers can show differences in cognitive strengths as early as in primary school. This raises new questions about whether we should learn our Apolipoprotein genotypes as children, if we are having trouble in school, despite the absence of a cure for Alzheimer's disease. Inverting that logic, I can't help but wonder if my excelling at school in the past means that I don't have an Apolipoprotein ε4 allele. Could we figure out the other genetic vulnerability factors and use that information to change our lifestyles early enough to compensate?

A combination of SNPs may result in a gene-on-gene interaction that creates risk for dementia, or it may be the SNP interacting with some environmental factor (e.g., exposure to secondhand cigarette smoke) that creates the risk. The way to look for those SNP effects across large populations is called genome-wide association study (GWAS), and we'll hear more about the hunt for those associations over the next 10 years. These scientists' work has led to a shift in focus from the human genome to the human "brainome."

In the summer of 2010, researchers identified a gene combination that runs counter to the longstanding lore that only ε4 lends risk for Alzheimer's: Apolipoprotein ε3, when present along with a variation of a separate gene called TOMM40, influences the size of brain regions that are most susceptible to the changes of Alzheimer's. Further examination will reveal whether this unfortunate combination is as highly associated with Alzheimer's disease manifesting outwardly as Apolipoprotein ε4 is.

Despite the fact that ε4 has remained a consistent finding among Alzheimer's disease populations, there are very many people with Alzheimer's disease who do *not* have an ε4 on board. We believe that they have come to Alzheimer's disease through other mechanisms, whether those are genetic mutations yet to be discovered or effects of the environment upon their genetically determined aging process.

When a particular SNP is reliably linked to a disease state, it is then called a mutation. So when used correctly, the label *mutation* implies that the direct genetic cause of a disease has been found. A good example of a genetic mutation with a strong causal link to a disease is the mutation in the gene for a protein called Huntingtin that leads to the development of Huntington's disease. In Huntington's disease, a series of triplets (the genetic equivalent of "yaddayaddayadda") disrupts the normal production of Huntingtin. The longer the series of triplets intruding onto an individual's gene, the more severe the symptoms.

With a first-degree relative who developed Alzheimer's disease, it would be reasonable for a person to wonder whether she has Apolipoprotein ε4. What would she then do with this information?

Dr. Margaret Lock, a professor emerita of social studies in medicine at McGill University, trained relatives of patients with Alzheimer's disease about genetic principles so that they might be able to understand the results of their genotype testing. Half of them were given the results of their testing, while the other half were not told what the results were. Researchers then monitored whether these study subjects changed their lifestyles in anticipation of higher susceptibility to Alzheimer's disease and also whether they retained the information about their genetic risk level.

Interestingly, many of the subjects who received the genotyping results could remember whether they were at higher risk compared to anyone else in the general population, but they did not remember the specifics of that information. Many felt annoyed knowing this information without being given any clear treatment recommendations to prevent Alzheimer's disease. There were no significant changes in these people's lifestyles. This latter point may have been related to the fact that usually volunteers for studies are highly motivated to keep themselves informed about the subject that they are participating in, and they may have already been following some of the current recommendations to reduce Alzheimer's disease risk.

Ah Quan was a second-degree relative to me. Ah Quan very likely had amyloid gumming up her arterial walls, which robbed them of their elasticity and led finally to the rupture that killed her. If not for Ah Quan's fatal hemorrhage, I might not suspect that I have Apolipoprotein $\varepsilon4$. But amyloid angiopathy is frequently associated with the individual's carrying at least one $\varepsilon4$ allele. Let's assume that she had one $\varepsilon4$ allele. My mother therefore has a 25% chance of having inherited an $\varepsilon4$ from her mother. This probability goes up if we assume that my grandfather was one of the approximately 15% of the general population who has an $\varepsilon4$. If each of my grandparents had one $\varepsilon4$, my mother's chance of getting one is 50% and of having two $\varepsilon4$ alleles is 25%. Does this mean that my mother will get Alzheimer's disease? She may not. In her eightieth year she sometimes complains that she's not as sharp as she used to be, but she is functioning at quite a high and independent level. She is teaching classes in Chinese brush painting and organizing art shows, keeping up with her girlfriends, and managing the household as she always did, and gets called back into service as a legal secretary for temporary work as much as she will consent to.

I saw Ah Quan a little less than annually, either in Honolulu (her home) or in Los Angeles at my parents' house. Ah Quan was held up as a high achiever, accomplished in big and little things that mattered. I have a vivid memory of how she was able to wrap gifts without having to use tape; the ends of the boxes were neatly turned in and every corner was sharp, so that each gift box was like an origami work. I still can't achieve that level of perfection and I utter a squeak of guilt every time I reach for the tape dispenser.

Whenever Ah Quan and my mother were together, they would fill their time with gardening or sewing projects. Or we would shuttle her to her favorite store for knitting goods, Super Yarn Mart. With her New England accent acquired from the missionaries in Hawai'i, it came out sounding funny to my ear: "Soopah YAHN Maht." Those were long trips, and we'd come back with skeins and skeins of fluorescent acrylics for scarves, booties, and gloves. I couldn't participate in those projects as a little girl, so my time to interact with Ah Quan was while we shared meals. My earliest memories of her were from the kitchen table. All that was asked of me was that I chew with my mouth shut. She had a gesture, thumb and forefinger touching and the circle they made rounding and flattening, to remind my brother and me that we were eating like stock animals. It was easy for me to measure up to those low requirements.

She also had a horrifying sneeze: It would start off sounding as if she'd just been stabbed in the back but ended more reassuringly in "-choo!" When they came to Los Angeles, my grandparents were on Hawai'i time, which meant that mealtimes were earlier, the house started making noise earlier, and, as with all visits of in-laws, there was stress between the primary couple. It was hard to understand why these old folks were so important that we had to go to such lengths, but this was probably my first exposure to the concept of respecting one's elders.

I don't have the Ah Quan sneeze, but I do have her voice, her smile canted to the right, her weakness for tropical flower leis, and her knack for correspondence. Has her propensity for Alzheimer's disease been transmitted to me as well?

Now that my parents are in their eighties, I am getting a better sense of what my own eighties might look like. I am happy to report that my father was last seen delighting extended family with a ukulele performance, the first time he's played in 14 years. I hope that "80 will be the new 60." In the meantime, all of the lifestyle factors that I can change for the better to reduce my potential risk of Alzheimer's disease, whether that risk is high due to Apolipoprotein ε4 or not, all happen to make good common sense and help to reduce identified risks for stroke and heart attack. There are many factors that contribute to one's overall risk profile for Alzheimer's disease, and that may be where we can rebalance the odds in our favor.

It is sobering to keep in mind that having a first-degree relative with Alzheimer's disease, regardless of ε4 status, triples a person's risk of getting Alzheimer's disease. That relates to the general population's decade-by-decade prevalence of Alzheimer's disease, or a proxy for the probability that one will have Alzheimer's disease. From age 60 to 65, the general prevalence of Alzheimer's disease is 2% to 2.5%. Those are pretty good odds! Even tripling this number yields less than a 10% chance of having Alzheimer's disease at age 60 to 65. However, this prevalence rate doubles with each five-year period. From age 65 to 70, we're looking at a 5% risk of getting Alzheimer's disease, without knowing any other information about parentage or genetic makeup or stroke risk factors; 5% multiplied by 3 is 15%, which is still a low percentage. Continuing in this fashion, by the time a person gets to his early eighties, there is a general Alzheimer's disease risk rate of 33%. This is when the tripling amounts to significant numbers: 33% multiplied by 3 is 99%, meaning that almost every one of those individuals 80 to 85 years old with a first-degree family member with Alzheimer's disease will follow suit.

The key to understanding which genetics lead most frequently to Alzheimer's disease has to include many SNPs beyond Apolipoprotein ε4. Significant contributions are made by SNPs that determine intelligence, memory function, how a person produces inflammatory responses, propensity to diabetes, the body's and brain's responsiveness to sex hormones, mood, fitness level for exercise, personality for social networking, dietary preferences, stroke risk factors, and longevity.

It follows that the contribution of genetics to Alzheimer's disease risk, although unalterable, is complex. The glass-half-empty view of this is that it will take a very long time to figure out which magic combination leads away from Alzheimer's disease. The glass-half-full view of this information is that even if we do have some genetically based risk factors for Alzheimer's disease, there are other things in our lives that we can alter over time to counterbalance those risks for developing this type of dementia. The degree to which this applies to other dementias is not yet clear. There is a more direct connection between genetic mutations and frontotemporal dementia than there is for Alzheimer's, but there are still many patients with frontotemporal dementia for whom a genetic link has not been found. There is plenty of room for research in this area, but the high prevalence of Alzheimer's, compared to other causes of dementia, makes the genes or SNPs for Alzheimer's easier to hunt for among populations.

Our grandparents did not have the benefit of this kind of

information. They had bigger worries at the time: world wars, the Great Depression. However, I am sure that part of their wish for us to have better lives would have included that we would make good use of information when it became available.

Along with our biological inheritance from our parents, another unchangeable aspect of our lives is race. The question of whether any particular races are more susceptible to or more protected from getting Alzheimer's disease is difficult to answer because of social, economic, and cultural differences that lead to different discovery rates. A particular segment of the population may seem to be protected against Alzheimer's disease if not all cases are diagnosed accurately or in a timely fashion, compared to a more medically inclined subset of the population. Cultural perceptions and expectations of cognitive function in elderly people can lead to an underdiagnosis of dementia or Alzheimer's disease.

I was tempted in the past to believe that Chinese-Americans were immune to Alzheimer's. During the earlier phases of my medical training, I worked in Chicago and San Diego, regions of the United States where Asian-Americans make up a small minority. It therefore did not seem strange to me that our dementia clinics did not feature Asian faces. When I started at UCLA, where most of the student body seems to be Asian or Middle Eastern in origin, it did strike me as odd and even encouraging that we did not treat the same demographic proportions in our dementia clinic. I was all set to gloat about my "Alzheimer's-preventive ancestry."

Exploring this hypothesis, I led screening for cognitive impairment and focus groups at Asian places of worship and seniors' centers. The results taught me that Asians *do* get

Alzheimer's disease. The reasons we didn't see many Chinese-American families at our clinic had to do with barriers to accurate and timely diagnosis, also known as diagnostic or referral bias. An example of a barrier to seeking medical attention for Alzheimer's disease is the social stigma that too often can be associated with dementia as a mental illness.

In traditional Asian cultures, epilepsy and psychosis were seen as indicators of something shameful or defective in a person. Not so unreasonably, they linked these disorders to something passed along in the family, such as fate or bad luck, as opposed to genes. The general reaction upon observing someone with this type of problem was to shun not only the patient but his entire family as well. With anyone labeled "crazy" in the family, other family members were also considered ill-fated and unmarriageable until further notice. The confusion and loss of self caused by dementia were lumped into the category of "Illnesses to Avoid," as if dementia could be contagious. Much of this stigmatization has changed with education, just as the attitude toward leprosy has, but it took many decades.

Once dementia is seen as an illness affecting the brain, a body part, people can feel much compassion and be there to help out, just as they might with a child suffering fever and chills from a temporary viral illness. In fact, emerging data suggest that a patient with Alzheimer's disease is feeling "puny" in the same way as those with flu symptoms. We are fairly tolerant of crabby, confused, or depleted attitudes among our friends who have been felled temporarily with a flu; it's harder to be so accepting for years at a time, but these newly discovered associations may help caregivers understand what the day feels like to a patient with Alzheimer's disease.

At this time, it is believed that, as with schizophrenia, the worldwide prevalence of Alzheimer's disease is about the same, regardless of race. There are certainly specific risk factors for Alzheimer's disease that correlate with race, however. Studies have shown that African-Americans and Hispanics have a higher stroke risk related to high blood pressure and diabetes. These certainly interact with all of the other complex Alzheimer's risks. Once these aspects of a racial population have been considered, there is no one race that has a higher risk of Alzheimer's outside of associated factors such as stroke risk.

In Chapter 2, I described a Chinese patient named Richard with frontotemporal dementia. His father had died at age 50 of the same illness. Richard's sister Nora was brought by her husband to my clinic a year after we diagnosed Richard. As in the case of Richard's family, the illness had encroached upon Nora and her husband's income-earning and parenting time. They had two teenaged daughters who were otherwise preparing to stretch their wings and leave the nest.

Nora was a professional woman who looked 20 years younger than her stated age. She was attractively dressed and had a warm, friendly smile. Her husband, Kirk, was the one to answer most of the questions in the interview. She would turn to him for the answers with a sweet smile that an observer would interpret as a shy or adoring deference to Kirk. But this was not her baseline personality: She had been very successful and independent. Kirk could not help but minimize Nora's symptoms. He was quick to observe and appreciate that she had not manifested the hot temper outbursts seen in Richard.

She had become increasingly quiet and passive, as well as child-like. Her open and ready smile, along with her youthful look, made her easy and pleasant to be around; on the street, strangers would not be able to tell that she could not dress herself or use a microwave oven.

Like Richard, Nora deteriorated rapidly. Within two years, a huge brain communication gap had disrupted her ability to perform intentional movements. When Kirk would tell her to raise her arm to put on a jacket, it was as if she could not hear him; he would have to raise her arm for her. She arrived at the latest appointment, again well coiffed, with perfect makeup, and in heels, but this was all now Kirk's handiwork. He had learned how to be her stylist and valet. Also like Richard and his wife, this couple were in their early fifties. Kirk quit his job in order to spend with Nora whatever time remained to her. This arrangement has been eating into their retirement savings, but Kirk reasons, "She's not going to need retirement money, and right now this is more important to me." Patients with late-onset dementia have already had time to build up their post-parenting social network, retirement budget, and long-term-care insurance plans. In many ways, the aging sector of the population makes plans to downsize responsibilities (household and financial) in anticipation of some level of disability, but middle-aged patients are caught completely off guard and rarely have resources at hand to address dementia.

More recently, Nora developed paroxysms of rage. She would suddenly snarl fearsomely, then settle back into her docile baseline. It was terrible to see. At first we worried that she'd been offended or injured, then felt the need to extinguish the agitated discomfort she was indicating. The tricky part was that these gestures were not necessarily expressions of frustration or pent-up anger, and they were generally not tied to what she was feeling emotionally. The disease had unhooked the link between feelings and facial expressions (grimace) and bodily gestures (shaking fists). Nora's illness has become more like Richard's initial symptoms of outrage.

Richard responded to medication for Parkinson's disease, in that his movement had loosened up, but he had been unable to communicate in sentences or even consistent single words. We had held a family meeting so that his four sons could work with our team. The social worker had explained how other families with children had a difficult time balancing school, helping at home, and understanding what was happening to their affected parent. Mindy and I found it hard to maintain our composure. It turned out that Richard's 10-year-old son had become the primary caregiver for his father during his mother's work hours. And the other kids at school, not understanding dementing illness at all, were more likely to ostracize the boys than to be able to offer support.

This was a family with two middle-aged siblings, Nora and Richard, affected with the same five-to-six-year prognosis as their father. If any of the third-generation family members were to become affected at the same age as Richard or Nora, it would be about 30 years in the future. We discussed the availability of genetic testing with both Richard's and Nora's spouses. Results of the testing are still pending, because new potential mutations were identified only this year, and the first round of genetic testing did not include them.

―――――――

One important point as I calculate my own risk of developing Alzheimer's disease is to recognize that my grandmother and I, despite our similarities, have led very different lives and therefore have accumulated different levels of risk. Ah Quan was born in Honolulu 60 years before me and spent most of her formative years in the home of missionaries on Judd Street. She survived two world wars, including the bombing of Pearl Harbor. I grew up in Los Angeles car culture, my high school friends and I dressed in the style of Boy George and the Eurythmics, and John Hughes's movies captured my teenaged milieu. Ah Quan had a 71-year-long relationship with her first sweetheart and had two children. I remained single and without children into my mid-life.

A woman who was 80 a decade ago—who lived through a first world war, came of age in the Great Depression, and survived a second world war—had an entirely different set of environmental exposures from a woman aged 40 now. Someone who is middle-aged now may have attained higher education and employment, enjoyed a more socially active lifestyle, and gotten more regular exercise. We are not the same 43-year-olds our grandmothers were! Does that lower our risk for Alzheimer's disease? Those who specialize in life-course epidemiology take such factors into account. Researcher Rachel Whitmer is based in Northern California at Kaiser Permanente, a health maintenance organization that has long advocated for geriatric care, and she has explored how smoking in mid-life may lead to dementia in late life. Alternatively, things that are healthy in one decade may not be as healthy for the same person later; for example, the use of estrogen supplementation.

Genetics may set a course for how the brain and body will function over a lifetime, but there are plenty of things people can do to change those directions.

6

SOMETIMES IT'S HARD
TO BE A WOMAN

My big brother once commented, "You run like a girl." He then ignored my snarky response to clarify more constructively that girls tend to swing their hands from left to right while on the run, which disrupts the intention of forward propulsion. It had sounded like a condemnation of my sex, but it turned out to be a helpful piece of counsel.

I hope that the observation "You get Alzheimer's like a girl" will lead to a better understanding of the disease. Statistics on the prevalence of Alzheimer's disease have consistently reported higher numbers in women than in men. The incidence rate (number of new cases per 100,000 persons over the course of a year) is not necessarily different between the sexes, but the longer survival of women results in a higher prevalence (the current number of living cases, no matter how new or old the diagnosis). Prevalence further increases when a large caseload survives with the diagnosis for a long time. Alzheimer's is the longest and slowest of the causes of dementia, lasting for up to 20 years, although the reported average duration is 13 years.

Since most caregivers of patients with Alzheimer's disease are women, the combination of direct assault and collateral damage makes this type of dementia of particular concern for women.

When the public is told that more women than men have Alzheimer's disease, many assume that the dementia is a severe manifestation of menopause. While fluctuations in sex hormone levels do affect cognition, it has been difficult to prove that Alzheimer's disease is the result of late-life estrogen deprivation.

Marjorie and her husband believed she had cognitive impairment related to menopause and hoped it was reversible. She had become increasingly disorganized. As a teacher in special education, she prided herself on assisting children whose autism severely limited their ability to learn in a regular classroom. She routinely traveled to her students' homes to provide individualized teaching, but now she had been increasingly late to those appointments. Toronto's traffic overwhelmed her, and her reports to her board of education, usually a model of clarity, were now opaque and tardy. She had an uneasy sense of unraveling. Her husband, Mark, had reassured her, suggesting it was probably menopause. At the start of her symptoms, she was 49, just entering menopause, and they ran an active household with three teenaged sons. It wasn't a surprise that she would feel distracted. But then she forgot to pick the boys up from hockey one night and wasn't particularly troubled about this uncharacteristic mistake. Mark became alarmed. At the same time, the school board had its concerns and insisted that Marjorie have a medical examination.

At my office, this now 52-year-old woman was quiet and would otherwise seem completely normal to an observer. Could her symptoms be related to depression, menopause, mid-life anxieties, or something irreversible, like dementia?

I began as I usually do, by explaining that we'd spend the next half hour testing her memory and other brain functions, to discover her strengths and weaknesses. She was inaccurate on counting backward from 100 by sevens and her performance did not improve when I switched to the easier task of counting backward by threes. She seemed to need more encouragement or prompting to complete long tasks than I would expect for someone of her age. She was a bit nervous about what we might find, so I wasn't sure whether to be concerned with her performance yet. On the other hand, I knew that she had administered these types of tests to her students and should have been very familiar with the instructions.

When I moved to a brief task that is a pattern recognition test, my heart sank, because she should definitely have picked up the trick to this test. I hold my palms up, with a silver dollar showing in my right hand. I put both hands behind my back, make movements that could be transferring the coin to my left hand, then present both hands closed in front of me. The patient has to guess—and it is a guess at this stage—where the coin is. At first I don't transfer it from the right hand, and I continue to present it in that hand until the patient chooses the right hand correctly three times in a row. Then I alternate hands, and when they catch on to that, I hold it twice in each hand before moving it. It's easier in practice than it sounds, since we mainly expect the patient to recognize the change in pattern, as opposed to reading the examiner's mind. Marjorie never caught on that the coin hadn't switched from the original hand. It was as if she were starting the task from scratch every time.

Her ability to remember short word lists well (*cat*, *apple*, *table*) implied that hers was not the memory problem one would expect for Alzheimer's disease. Instead, she was having trouble juggling information mentally, and organizing commands into action. When asked to copy a sequence of three hand movements, she could say, "Flat, fist, edge," accurately, but her hand was not obeying.

Solving mathematical problems in her head was difficult; "If you pay for four cans of pop that cost forty cents each with a five-dollar bill, how much change should you get back?" was unsolvable among all the details. But she was able to perform simple arithmetic in her head when prompted for one solution at a time ("How much is four times forty?"). She could make a good copy of most figures (a cube, two pentagons that overlap at one corner). But everything was done slowly and without confidence.

At the end of the visit, we brought Mark back into the room so that I could discuss my concerns with them both. His face fell as I confirmed his fear that something was going wrong in Marjorie's brain. I stated that the pattern of difficulties revealed by the tests was not due to depression, and the severity of problems went beyond menopausal cognitive impairment.

Two types of dementia are possible for people in their fifties: Marjorie might have frontotemporal dementia or Alzheimer's disease, albeit a form that was starting much earlier in her life than most people associate with the illness. Marjorie seemed to absorb this pronouncement with a measure of indifference. Mark, on the other hand, was distraught. After hearing about each test we planned, he would ask, "What if it comes out normal? Won't that mean you're wrong?"

The day after their first clinic visit, Mark needed me to repeat my explanation of how I had come to the conclusion that his wife had an irreversible brain condition called dementia. He had read through the material we had given him about the disease the day before, and by the end of the phone call, he agreed that the description fit with Marjorie's behavior of the last three years. But part of his job as husband and caregiver was to make sure that every other possibility had been considered and ruled out. I repeated the rationale for ordering two types of brain scans to confirm this terrible diagnosis, and we went through the algorithms of what normal and abnormal results of either study would indicate about the diagnosis.

It was easiest to conclude the conversation by saying that I hoped I would be wrong. I told him that if this was not a form of dementia, I would be hard-pressed to make another diagnosis; the brain scans would help us to rule out brain tumor or some odd form of slowly advancing disease.

Three weeks later, the first of the two brain scans had been completed, yet the results were not conclusive. The radiologist's report was phrased ambiguously. In addition to categorizing the scan as a "Normal MRI of [the] brain," he stated that Marjorie's brain appeared "reasonably well-preserved." Reading between the lines, I understood this to mean that the brain looked fairly normal, and without knowing that this person has cognitive and behavioral changes, the scan would be read as "within normal limits." But the range of normal is wide, and the radiologist was telling me in his own way that the brain was just this side of showing some abnormal shrinkage.

I had promised Mark that I would relay the imaging results as soon as they were faxed to my clinic, but I knew he would ask if I had seen the scans with my own eyes. An abnormal MRI would prove the diagnosis, but the converse was not true: A "normal" MRI would not rule out the dementia diagnosis for Marjorie, since early in the illness, the structure of the brain may remain grossly unchanged. We would get more sensitive information from the second brain scan, called a SPECT scan, which detects changes in blood flow activity patterns that can predate volume loss. Unfortunately, we would have to wait two months to perform that more sensitive test. Somehow, Mark and Marjorie got through the Christmas holidays with the specter of a diagnosis in the background. When the results of the SPECT scan arrived, the findings were consistent with early-onset Alzheimer's disease.

Months later, Marjorie has responded slightly to the same medication given to much older patients with Alzheimer's disease. She speaks optimistically of how long she hopes it will hold. She is participating in an Alzheimer Society of Toronto support group for patients who are in an early stage of Alzheimer's disease. Mark brought the children in to the Memory Clinic to discuss their mother's condition and what they can expect in the next couple of years. They make a tall, wholesome-looking family, and I anticipate that the children will feel conflicted, as they prepare for university studies, about whether they should stay close to home to help care for their mother or go farther away, so that they can expend more energy moving their lives forward. Mark and Marjorie are lucky to have children who are old enough to handle their own basic care and who have friendships that will see them through Marjorie's decline.

When Ah Quan was in her forties, *Alzheimer's disease* was not a household term. Most illnesses were not talked about. Instead, the newspapers of the 1950s reported which celebrities had sailed into Honolulu Harbor, what the role of American military bases was in the Korean War, and how Hawai'i had bid for statehood. The ladies' section of the newspaper was adorned with pictures of brides-to-be and featured many "quick and easy" recipes, some of which encouraged the use of eggs for all three meals. There were a few public service announcements about what to do in case of a nuclear attack. The medical column addressed topics such as vitamin B12 deficiencies, nail biting, and the safety of vaccinations for children. Menopausal issues were not mentioned at all. Since then, menopause has become a regular topic of conversation among men and women in mid-life, especially in the context of their expectations of aging.

Women experience menopause at about age 50, with the typical onset ranging between ages 40 and 60. The decline of estrogen production during menopause has been suspected of being a trigger for Alzheimer's disease occurring in women. Is the disappearance of estrogen from the system a trigger for the deposition of amyloid or formation of tangles? I had been following the literature on estrogen supplementation and menopause, for my mother's sake, after a rather dramatic incident when I was a first-year medical student. I received a phone call from a friend in Los Angeles, my hometown, who asked, somewhat nervously, about my mother's health. Mom had been in a small fender-bender a month prior, but there had been no injuries, so I wondered aloud why he was asking. He suggested that I check in with my father.

My parents are of the generation that considers long-distance phone calls a luxury, so my father was surprised to be called, particularly while he was working at his dental practice. He did not volunteer any information until I mentioned my friend's inquiry. "Oh, that ...," he began reticently. "Well ..., your mother had a fall." And then it all tumbled out of him in a terrible, jarring description. She had stumbled and fallen in the garage, then a big piece of glass had toppled away from its usual supporting wall to shatter on top of her. She'd lain in the same spot for three hours, waiting for him to come home from work. Mom had a broken wrist, and her femur was so severely fractured that she would need a hip replacement.

Are you wincing while reading this? I'm wincing while writing it, decades later! I caught the next flight to Los Angeles. The orthopedic surgeon reported to us in the waiting room that the operation revealed Mom's bones to have aged 25 years faster than the rest of her body, due to osteoporosis. This launched me into a literature review of estrogen supplementation and risks for osteoporosis. I learned with a small degree of complacency that my swimming habit throughout medical school should provide some degree of protection against osteoporosis. My height, well above five feet, was also in my favor, but Asian women tend to be bird-boned. I learned then about the different formulations of estrogens, and that taking unopposed estrogen (without progesterone) brought on more risks than benefits. While the general populace understands the relationship between low levels of estrogen and osteoporosis, confusion reigns when it comes to the effects of estrogen on the brain.

Studies conducted to investigate whether hormone supplementation can protect against Alzheimer's disease have been contradictory. Earlier in life, some women complain that they are less able to sustain concentration or have word-finding difficulties at a particular point in pregnancy. Most of them regain their baseline abilities after they've settled into motherhood and reverted to a decent sleep pattern.

Following on the logic that childbearing changes hormonal levels drastically, epidemiologists have explored whether having more children increases or decreases the risk of getting Alzheimer's disease. Fertility (having one child, more than two, or none) has not been correlated with Alzheimer's disease risk. Similar cognitive complaints can re-emerge at the time of menopause. These associations between estrogen levels and memory loss have created great intrigue but few solid answers.

In addition, pregnancy and menopause have both been associated with mood swings. Just think of what a hot-button issue it is when a woman's partner muses out loud that premenstrual syndrome is the cause of their argument. Emotions, of course, have an impact on cognition that is difficult to treat as a separate issue when one considers premenstrual syndrome.

The Baltimore Longitudinal Study of Aging indicated that women who used hormonal supplementation, whether for contraception or the treatment of menopausal symptoms, seemed to have a lower risk ratio for Alzheimer's disease. But it was the adverse effects of taking estrogens that closed down the ensuing preventive drug trials. It is hard to ignore serious adverse events like uterine cancer, stroke, heart attack, *and* cognitive impairment when they occur more frequently in the group taking hormone supplements. Biochemists argue that the wrong formulation of estrogens was administered in these studies. Certainly, the area warrants more research. (Google "WHIMS," which stands for Women's Health Initiative Memory Study, for ongoing reports from this study.)

Conclusions from prior studies on aging women may not apply to my situation. A major difference between my age cohort and women of Ah Quan's generation is the use of oral contraceptives. Unlike today's high school girls who regularly take birth control pills for painful menstruation as well as birth control, Ah Quan was not exposed to pharmacologic estrogen supplementation. Bench research (that involving test tubes in a lab, but not necessarily clinical trials done on humans) has shown that higher estrogen levels—or perhaps creating more steady levels of estrogen with the Pill over the reproductive years—has effects on the brain. Neurons sprout more connections with each other, for instance. Has that offered an advantage for women of my generation? Does it add to cognitive reserve to decrease future vulnerability? One can hope, but it is still unclear.

For the cohort of women who have already initiated hormonal oral contraception, the question has changed from "Should I use the Pill?" to "When is the right time to stop using it?" Or is it better to go with a non-hormonal alternative, such as tubal ligation after a certain age? We don't know yet. Women should discuss the benefits and risks of hormonal contraception or supplementation with their doctors. Those lucky enough not to have high blood pressure, obesity, or high cholesterol and who don't smoke can worry less about prolonged hormonal contraceptive use. The average monthly probability of conception declines by half in most women as they hit their mid-forties, yet even women during perimenopause still need effective contraception. Some of the other benefits of hormonal contraception might include correction of menstrual cycle abnormalities, or protection against severe acne, osteoporosis, endometriosis, and colorectal cancer. Some benefits are positively correlated with the duration of use, and those benefits may extend 10 years or more after stopping the Pill.

The list of drawbacks to hormonal supplementation after menopause is long: increased risk of some but not other types of gynecological cancer, unwanted blood clotting, migraine headache, uterine cancer, stroke, heart attack, *and* cognitive impairment. The latest consensus on this subject is that hormonal supplementation in a woman's mid-life (ages 40 to 60) may be beneficial, while supplementation in late life (over 60, some say over 70) is actually detrimental. That conclusion supports the idea that timing can have as much impact as the particular formulation of estrogen delivered. There has been no clear superiority shown among topical, oral, or herbally-based preparations.

In response, a field of study has emerged on the effects of sex hormones on the brain at different stages of life, including: adolescence; the childbearing years and their related major fluctuations in hormones; the postpartum period when women complain that they are having word-finding problems or even memory problems (most of which resolve spontaneously); and then perimenopause and its multimillion-dollar question of whether hormone replacement is beneficial for perimenopausal women, and if so, in which formulations of estrogen and progesterone.

Even if we can keep in mind that the incidence of Alzheimer's disease is the same for men and women, one cellular finding implicates Alzheimer's disease with the female sex. The abnormal protein collections seen in brains from patients who had dementia accumulate at least in part due to impaired function of the mitochondrion, which is important as the energy processor and fuel manager for each cell. When the mitochondrion isn't working correctly, the cell can't operate well. The DNA used for the body's mitochondria (the plural of *mitochondrion*) comes *only from the mother*. Paternal DNA for the mitochondria is ignored in both male and female anatomy. Despite this fact, it has not been proven that children of a mother with Alzheimer's disease are more at risk than children of a father with Alzheimer's disease. Mitochondrial function is probably one contributing factor as to whether someone will manifest dementia in later life. One can imagine the combined difficulty of carrying Apolipoprotein ε4 alleles, having DNA for mitochondria that do not age well, and attaining a low educational level as accumulated risk factors for Alzheimer's disease.

It is natural to assume that differences between the sexes are caused by hormones. It is not so straightforward, though, to reason that women live longer than men because of estrogen, since estrogen levels drop after menopause. Because the timing of hormone release varies over a lifespan, any causal relationships that may exist between hormones and risk for late-life dementia will remain unclear until data from throughout the lifespan have been collected and analyzed. The majority of patients living with Alzheimer's are women, and research thus far has shown that the relationship between estrogen and brain function is influenced by many other aspects of life, ranging from cognitive reserve to genetics.

Hormones are also associated with emotion, mood, and stress, and each of these can create serious vulnerability to Alzheimer's disease, regardless of sex.

MANAGE YOUR STRESS
BEFORE IT MANAGES YOU

Have you ever noticed that people who work long, hard hours year-round can be laid low with a virus as soon as they go on vacation? That focus on stressful work activity without maintaining a balance—in diet, in other aspects of life—takes its toll on the immune system. Stress can also increase one's risk for developing dementia. When the brain perceives stress, it signals the release of cortisol from the adrenal glands. Cortisol is useful for getting us through brief and necessary rough patches of life, but chronically dosed from within, cortisol keeps blood pressure high, deposits fat around the waist, and promotes heartburn and gastric ulcers.

Another adverse effect of the chronic release of cortisol, which is harder to see until it is too late, is shrinkage of the hippocampus, the part of the brain that we rely upon for the retention of new information. One of my favorite university professors spent decades studying the effects of stress on baboons. Dr. Robert Sapolsky spent summers observing East African baboon troop hierarchies and taking blood samples to characterize each baboon's stress hormone levels. Part of what he learned from his research is that high release of cortisol—which in the baboons' case stemmed from sitting at the bottom of the baboon pecking order—can shrink the hippocampus. This happens in humans as well. The hippocampus is the area of the brain, deep and on the underside, that serves as a filing system for incoming information. No hippocampus, no new memories. Imagine the mind being stuck at one point of a life history but living each day fairly normally otherwise. The person could still cook, drive a car, and send email but would not remember much about these activities the next day. The movie *50 First Dates* used this type of amnesia as an effective romantic plot device: Adam Sandler had to win Drew Barrymore's heart over and over again every day.

Alzheimer's disease entails more than just short-term memory loss like this, but the hippocampus and its neighbor-hood are the epicenter of the pathological changes. Whatever a person can do to protect the hippocampus from excessive stress and keep it robustly connected to the rest of the brain's memory processing hubs can help stave off Alzheimer's disease.

We all require stimulation to enhance the brain's plasticity, but we also require just the right amount of cortisol-inducing activity and not too much. We all understand the risks of job burnout, but if my job were going to result in brain-out, it wouldn't be worth it. Dr. Sapolsky has learned that lowering stress and corticosteroid levels allows the hippocampal region to recover size and function. "We are not getting our ulcers being chased by saber-tooth tigers, we're inventing our social stressors—and if some baboons are good at dealing with this, we should be able to as well," he writes. "Insofar as we're smart enough to have invented this stuff and stupid enough to fall for it, we have the potential to be wise enough to keep the stuff in perspective." Dr. Sapolsky does not accept any invitations to speak at conferences unless he can be home in time to tuck his children into bed. He draws a thick line to let everyone know where his home life needs to be balanced against his professional life, and that's exemplary.

I feel I owe it to my hippocampi—yes, there is one on the left and another on the right side of the brain—to keep them as plump as I can. Women of the last few generations have struggled with self-induced expectations that we can Do It All. In gratitude for the struggle of generations before us, we want to achieve right alongside men. And we also want reproductive freedom—not just to determine the time to have children, but also to decide whether we keep our jobs while we raise our children. Sadly, it is the rare mother who feels she is doing a terrific job both at work and at home. Far too many of us feel stretched thin, either missing in action from the extended workday (earning the medical boys' club epithet of "weak tinkler") or working those long hours and leaving the children's supervision to someone else ("absentee mother!"). And, oh yes, is there any time budgeted for nurturing a relationship with a significant other?

In generations preceding mine, the couple expected to divide the labor. A father figure was meant to go out and be the breadwinner, engaging with family mostly at bedtime and on weekends, while the mother was charged with tending the household and raising the children. Even if she did work outside of the home, it was clear to all that her family life came first.

In today's double-income households, neither breadwinner is a full-time parent. If an extraterrestrial visitor were to visit children in my neighborhood, he might report back that the only fertile humans seem to be young women from the Philippines (who are employed as nannies).

When I see friends struggling as single parents, I have respect for their ability to get it all done, but I know that their productivity comes at the expense of sleep or quality time with children or looking competitive for promotion. This kind of arrangement doesn't work unless there's help, but I think many of my women friends don't feel comfortable about asking for help, whether at work or at home.

That is just one type of stress. The emotional stress of illness can be profound, as is the stress of taking care of someone who has a chronic illness. And accumulated stress leads to higher risk of brain dysfunction later in life.

Most people can readily recognize whether they have a lot of stress in their lives. And some people reach for readily accessible "self-medication" for stress, in the form of alcohol, recreational drugs, or tobacco. In my grandmother's newsletter and newspapers of the early 1960s, the health hazards of smoking had just come under debate, being not yet fully proven or acknowledged. People were slow to understand that smoking might be dangerous. Mark Waters, a journalist, wrote his own poignant obituary before dying of lung cancer. On the day I was born in 1966, the *Honolulu Star-Bulletin* published his piece, entitled, "I Met My Killer 42 Years Ago." Smoking is a risk factor for heart disease, heart attack, and high blood pressure; all of these are themselves risk factors for stroke. Any of those illnesses incurs higher risk for dementia, especially vascular dementia. One study reported that smoking doubles one's risk for dementia, and no one can absolutely predict that lung cancer will kill someone before dementia develops. Even if smokers are willing to take their chances with dementia in order to keep smoking, they might consider the effects on family and friends who will have to become their caregivers in the event that smoking causes a terminal illness, whether cancer or dementia.

Apart from corticosteroid toxicity, stress can trigger other conditions, such as migraine headache, diabetic complications, or an outbreak of herpes. I was startled one morning after a busy night on-call to experience the same symptoms as the last patient I had admitted through the emergency room. She'd complained of visual changes that might have been a stroke. On closer questioning, I recognized that she was describing the scintillations (sparkly lights) and scotomas (blind spots) that mark the onset of a migraine headache. She was older than usual for a first-time migraine, but we treated her for migraine and she improved. I woke up in my call-room a few hours later, rumpled in scrubs and tired but grateful to have been allowed to sleep at all. I was preparing to introduce the Neurology Rounds speaker when I noticed flashing, sparkly lights in the right side of my visual field.

I thought it was odd, but I was too distracted to think more about it. After introducing the speaker, I finally noticed a blind spot with interspersed blinking flashers on the right side of my vision. Recalling the questions I'd put to the previous night's patient, I closed one eye, then the other. The visual change, called an aura, was happening in both eyes, not just one. That meant I wasn't likely to be suffering the retinal detachment that we extremely nearsighted folks (high myopes) fear. Good news. But could I be having my first migraine with aura fewer than 12 hours after talking to a woman who was admitted to hospital with her first migraine with aura?

At first I was a little disappointed with my lack of originality, but then was morbidly fascinated with the visual disturbance—how interesting! My mind's eye scrolled down to the part of the "Migraine Headache" chapter that states, "The visual aura often ends in twenty minutes, to be followed by a dull, unilateral headache." Unlike most of my patients, I had read the textbook, and the headache came, right on schedule. Since then, my migraines have come during times of major stress. Even if I think I can tough out high-stress situations, the recurrence of blind spots and headaches serves as my reality check. Because women (not men) over age 45 who suffer weekly migraine have greater odds of suffering a stroke, I have even more incentive to keep stress (and therefore the migraines) at bay. I want to avoid migraines, and I want to avoid Alzheimer's disease! Another enticement to control stress is that, much like with smoking, quitting the harmful habit can yield positive results within months.

Adjusting the amount of time and energy spent on a stressful activity such as caregiving can be difficult. My parents taught my brother and me to consider the needs of others first. Compassion is important, but it takes skill to stop short of overextending oneself.

My friend Bill once gave me a pendant carved out of red coral. He sent it in a box accompanied by an explanation: The figure pictured was Quan Yin, the Chinese version of the bodhisattva for compassion, and Bill said I reminded him of her. The brief description recounted how Quan Yin was so compassionate that she refused to advance to the most enlightened state until everyone else in the world had gone ahead of her. She is, of course, still waiting.

I was at first touched and flattered by the compliment. My curiosity about this character from the Buddhist canon led me to the library at the Metropolitan Museum of Art, which holds an extensive Hindu sculpture collection. After extensive reading, I reformed my opinion: Quan Yin may well rank as the Supreme Co-Dependent of the Universe! She is often depicted in sculpture as having a thousand arms, and on each of those thousand palms is an eye for her (him, in some cultures) to perceive suffering throughout the world. Tireless? You bet! Always ready to hear about anyone's suffering. Comes in two modes: the Gentle, Nonjudgmental Listener, and the Warrior to avenge suffering. I felt worn out just reading about it. These are wonderful expectations for a deity, but I was just getting to the middle of my life and feeling depleted. For regular mortals, if compassion is practiced without wisdom, the well can run dry; resentful feelings burble up and can undercut the joy that ought to accompany the compassionate act.

Equanimity and compassion tempered by wisdom are two of Buddhism's Four Intentions. Another is loving kindness. Loving kindness is the practice of helping others to feel safe, loved, healthy, and at ease. This is a key to success as a caregiver, whether a person is a formally trained health worker or an untrained family member. One manifestation of loving kindness that is very difficult for family members to practice is forgiving the patient for no longer being able to fulfill former roles. The spouse who cannot accept that her husband is no longer capable of encouraging or comforting her due to his dementia has to bear the burden of unresolved feelings of neglect. That in turn impedes her from finding new ways to have her emotional needs met. This compounds the amount of stress she feels as a care provider. I think marriages that have lasted happily for decades are operating on some version of this unconditional loving kindness, in which we wish the other person to feel safe, loved, healthy, and at ease. It is a profoundly solid foundation for a relationship, regardless of the turns it must take.

In my practice, I meet couples who have been together for a lifetime, and it is moving to be around the kind of love that has weathered so gracefully. Even after spoken language had deteriorated between Helen and Joe, I saw them sitting side by side at an appointment, probably dreading what I would tell them about how much Helen's Alzheimer's disease has worsened, or that I would have to repeat for the fourth time in two years that there is still no cure available, no new medication to try. Helen was not able to understand the specifics of my comments anymore, but she understood the context of being in a doctor's office, and that she was the subject of the visit. But then her flat expression would warm into a smile whenever she felt Joe lean ever so slightly against her. There was a physical sign of relaxation when they held hands to leave the room. They had a long history together as ballroom dancers, and when they took each other's hands to leave, they seemed to glide away. Joe was content knowing that his presence was such a comfort to Helen, and her acknowledgment of his role in her life was in turn a comfort to him. When marriages continue to work despite the spectre of dementia, those very subtle and timeworn displays of affection and kindness are wonderful to behold.

The most important thing I've learned about loving kindness is that it begins with wishing *oneself* to be feeling safe, loved, and healthy, and living with ease. Then each of us extends that wish to others around us, and if it's easier to start with familiar people, that's fine. The goal is to be able to make that wish on behalf of all living things. It's okay and highly recommended to start with oneself, not others.

One study concluded that caregivers of patients with dementia were at a higher risk of developing dementia themselves. This most likely has to do with the unrelenting stress of being a caregiver. But too often that stress is self-induced. It never fails to surprise me how so few caregivers feel that they deserve some respite or leisure time. Leisure time is for managing stress, and it may be a crucial factor in the caregiver's own vulnerability to Alzheimer's or other dementias, like the type caused by stroke. While we cannot always avoid negative situations or harm, we can work on how that harm affects how we perceive the world and ourselves in it. Meditation or mindfulness practices can help a person make that perceptual shift.

With dementia, the demands on the caregiver can last for years. The landscape is always shifting, and the disease unfolds against the backdrop of personal loss. A long-term personal relationship with someone means there is also a shared history. Each partner has taken on roles in the other's life, and even if those roles may have shifted over time, there is still a clear "job description" that is filled or adjusted to meet both people's needs. When one partner suffers cognitive losses or behavioral and personality alterations, some of those aspects of the relationship may remain, while others are lost. The caregiver may still feel connected to the patient, with a growing role as someone who needs to safeguard the other. The patient, on the other hand, is absolved gradually of most or all duties.

The balance has been upset, and most caregivers find too late that their own needs have not been met. They might wonder, "Where is the loving kindness for me?" Sometimes they intentionally put off the practice of loving kindness for themselves, holding their breath until the end of the dementia. But dementias can last for as long as 20 years, too long to delay gratification of one's needs. At worst, a caregiver will feel trapped and resentful of the patient and others who are not contributing to care. One of the major themes of education in our clinic is the idea of pacing—making time for oneself amid the caregiving duties. This almost always requires that the caregiver share the experience with others.

One caregiver who stands out for me is Brian, whose wife, Wendy, has frontotemporal dementia. Her language abilities have declined rapidly over the past year. She used to be able to have conversations with the occasional interruptions of "Cute" and other compliments tossed in haphazardly. Then she was reduced to using pat phrases, and now she uses very little speech at all. Her illness has made her constantly euphoric, despite her inability to organize or perform basic activities of daily living. Brian quickly mastered the art of recruiting concerned family and friends to Wendy's side by educating them. He distributed this email update before taking Wendy to a family reunion:

Making Connections
As Wendy's disease progresses, we will see less communication initiated by her. She will appear to be distant and non-respon-sive to greetings and questions posed to her. However, she still

seeks "connection" with her family and friends in her own way. You have to help make that happen! She is not hard of hearing, just unresponsive, so speak in a clear, normal voice. She will not answer most questions with more than a "yes" or "no," or "maybe yes" or "maybe no." If you ask questions that can be answered with yes or no, she will usually continue to connect with you. She likes to walk, but must always be with someone unless she is in the house ... even then keep an eye on her since she is elusive as a five-year-old. She is an "observer": she may stare at you, perhaps because she is recalling something about you, or something about you fascinates her (you might get a face rub, a head rub, or a casual touch of something on your clothes). When she eats, you must make sure that she has small portions. If you are next to her, offer to cut up some pieces so that she can eat. She doesn't use a knife. Sometimes Wendy will take your hand or lightly touch your arms or cheeks. Don't be alarmed ... some of her connections are made through touch; she fondly remembers her physical connection with you. She just can't tell you this in words so she is reaching out to you!

Those instructions were written with loving kindness and tell the readers how to help Wendy feel loved and safe in their company. This is a great way to describe the patient and her caregiver's needs. And it met with success.

There's a shortlist for caregivers to consider for themselves, too. At the end of the day, ask yourself:

- Did I achieve everything on the checklist for the patient?

- Was I able to do something for him or her?
- How am I doing? Am I safe, healthy, happy, and feeling loved?

Doing something for the patient may include assisting in eating a meal or performing some other activity of daily living with or for her. Sometimes the greatest thing a person can do for the patient is to be with her quietly and without expectations, that is, to have quality time together. This does not require much knowledge of the patient or skillful conversation. We see so many caregivers pushing themselves and the patients into irritated states, despite the best of intentions. While it is true that stimulation may be good for the brain, rehearsing patients on mental status tests that we use in the office to gauge cognitive impairment or prompting patients to recall stories can actually cause distress. The patient may well understand that she is not performing to expectation, but that may be the best she can do. And caregivers need to be informed by the health care team at what point the rehearsals do not lead to cognitive maintenance. Instead, the focus should be on setting the patient up for success and allowing that person to feel accepted and valued as she is. Ah Quan's parting advice on relationships was, "Be kind to each other." The practice of loving kindness entails letting go of former expectations. Instead of clinging to a less painful past, caregivers can strive for equanimity to appreciate whatever meaningful interaction can be brought to each day.

It takes a certain amount of grace and creativity to find the poetry within the broken narrative that is dementia. The loss of a person's ability to tell his own story is tragic, if a linear trajectory is the only workable form of communication. But in poetry, there is room for flexibility of interpretation—imagery, gesture, and metaphor have to fill in. How great it is when the caregiver or friend visiting the patient can meet him or her halfway in enjoying an interaction that is mostly improvised, and that has no particular agenda, other than perhaps bringing some sense of play and lightness into the day.

I recently attended a concert by Bobby McFerrin, where he walked onto the stage with just a chair and a bottle of water. Bobby McFerrin is able, through a keen sense of playfulness, to transform himself into a musical instrument, and by extension, everything he touches or interacts with also becomes a musical instrument, including the audience. He began the evening with several improvised songs—there were no recognizable lyrics. If there were any words, there were only two or three which did not tell any particular story. All the same, we were enchanted. After the first 20 minutes, he addressed the audience and I was shocked, despite myself, to recognize a normal man's speaking voice coming from him. Up until that moment, it was easy to believe that he was something other than a regular person, magically able to connect with us nonverbally.

I began to think of this as an example of the best a caregiver might be able to achieve in enjoying time with a patient who has lost language or coherence. If we can let go of our expectation that the other person should follow a logical stream of thought, with the usual pauses for turn-taking in conversation, and if we can instead take up the challenge of improvising how we spend time with the patient, there will be more opportunity for the patient to connect with us.

Bobby McFerrin will often invite audience members onto the stage to perform with him in an improvisational exercise. When he called for some people to dance up on stage, I answered the call to come out and play. We had never met before; he did not know what my previous dance training has been, and given his repertoire of musical talents, I had to be ready for anything. I had nothing to lose and only a fun, memorable experience to gain. What ensued probably lasted for less than two minutes, but it was exhilarating. I could tell he was modulating to different styles of music, as he saw how I was moving, whether I was playing to the audience or to him, or just getting tangled up in the very long sleeves of my sweater. I changed my movement with the rhythm, tempo, or emotional style of what I was hearing. We weren't competing with each other and we were just, within the very loose guidelines of improvisation, exploring what we could do together.

Gail Elliot of DementiAbility, a consulting firm for caregivers who seek feasible and meaningful activities for patients with dementia, has introduced me to Montessori methods that bring that improvisational attitude to working with patients who have dementia. The Montessori name may ring familiar as a popular schooling philosophy that advances young children through grade school with curricula individualized to their interests, motivation, and strengths. Optimally, this method also provides flexibility to accommodate both budding bookworms who like to sit and the more restless, "kinetic" learner. Gail's tailored activities and materials allow caregivers to interact with patients at whatever level those patients can achieve on a given day. Each activity has several levels of difficulty, and so a patient might be able to place colored blocks on top of a template or go all the way to translating a flat drawing into something built out of the same blocks. In yoga, the instructor will demonstrate a position that helps stretch the legs, and then there are additional prompts for those students in the room who are more flexible and can add a twist or more depth to the same pose. The yoga instructor and the family member practicing Montessori methods encourage achievement each day, but only "as far as your practice takes you today," implying that participation is perfectly fine as a goal, as opposed to being the best in the room.

It is possible and even imperative for caregiver–patient interactions to be open and playful. But first it requires letting go of expectations of the patient's former abilities, letting go of the shared history that shaped those expectations over many years. I will not delude myself that this is easy to do, but I urge caregivers to make an effort to have one interaction like this each day with the patient, however brief. The idea is to have quality time together, to underscore or acknowledge that joy is an important part of life and is integral to the feelings of safety, health, and being loved.

While I am not formally trained to be a family counselor, I regularly recognize caregivers who are exceedingly hard on themselves. Unless the caregiver has had some medical training, he or she frequently feels inadequate or feels personally responsible for progression of illness in the patient. Even if physical needs are being met, there is always time for doubting whether the family has done enough to research better treatments, better doctors, or better resources. (See the Appendices for tips on how to read about the latest findings critically and make decisions about research participation.)

Self-esteem is also linked to Alzheimer's risk. People experience a more beneficial cortisol production rate when self-esteem is high. That comfortable sense of self varies among individuals and is affected by life's experiences and by genetic makeup. Regardless of emotional or spiritual background, one can develop skills in appreciating the joyful aspects of life and practicing a compassionate outlook with equal concern for self and others.

Raising one's self-esteem enhances something referred to as the "locus of control." For example, it doesn't matter if others believe someone to be the best of caregivers if he still feels resentful for not having time to take care of himself. He might start trying to live up to his reputation instead of attending to his own needs. In that case, the locus of control is off-center. Balancing out self-care and actions that merit praise from others is critical to one's perception of how life is going. Evidence shows that increasing self-esteem scores has an additional payoff in decreasing the amount of cortisol the brain releases in response to unavoidable stress.

Caregivers need to watch out for loss of self-esteem as fallout from the daily stress. There is also a very high incidence of depression among caregivers. Where there is a sense of loss, hopelessness, and guilt, depression is likely to arise. Having depressive episodes in mid-life and then again in late life increases the risk of developing dementia, independent of familial risk factors. It is not so clear yet whether treating the depression thoroughly enough to avoid the recurrence in late life can prevent or delay dementia onset. Depression among caregivers can be treated, and my nurse and I will always encourage caregivers who are showing signs of hopelessness and helplessness to get counseling or seek help from psychiatrists to manage this mood disorder.

There are many allied organizations dedicated to helping caregivers, both during active caregiving and afterward. The Alzheimer's Association of the United States and the Alzheimer Society of Canada were founded to provide help to caregivers. The original slogan of the Alzheimer's Association was, "Someone to stand by you," and the emphasis was on making sure that caregivers had support during the long course of dementia. As the organization grew and caregiver support groups led by social workers or others became widely available, the focus shifted to making sure that health care professionals and public service providers, such as emergency medical service personnel and police officers, were educated about dementia. One of the most important resources established in both countries is the identification network to locate a patient who has wandered from a day program or home, called "Safe Return" in the United States and "Safely Home" in Canada. Most recently, the Alzheimer's Association has become a major fundraiser for research; the byline for both the Alzheimer's Association and the Alzheimer Society of Canada is now, "Our vision is a world without Alzheimer's disease." Both organizations provide counseling services to formal and informal caregivers and understand that they have an important role to play in advancing research.

Caregivers find some comfort in commiseration, but they also form a very active advocacy group that is keen to find the cure. Alzheimer's associations all over the world coordinate resources and share educational materials in various languages. The organizations sponsor two international conferences: the Alzheimer Association International Conference® meets in July and is attended by many of us in scientists; the Alzheimer Disease International (ADI) conference is aimed more at provision of social services and administration of long-term-care facilities. Caregivers may find ADI useful to attend, especially if they have an interest in political advocacy.

The executive director of the Alzheimer's Association chapter in Philadelphia, Helen-Ann Comstock, realized halfway through the course of her husband's illness that he did not, in fact, have Alzheimer's disease but rather frontotemporal dementia. She quickly learned that there were no resources for caregivers of patients with frontotemporal dementia, and thus the Association for Frontotemporal Degeneration was born in 2002. Meanwhile, in the United Kingdom, caregivers of people with dementia with Lewy bodies united their forces in 2003; the organization expanded to North America and is now headquartered in the United States.

With access to the internet, any of these groups is accessible to all caregivers. Mary Mittelman of New York University, whose research has focused on caregiver support, has steadily reported evidence that counseling home caregivers (mostly spouses), even if that help is only provided by telephone, leads to better quality of life for both the caregivers and patients with dementia. Her recent systematic review of the literature also reports that multi-component caregiver support delays institutionalization and improves patient behavior.

Due to the long-term nature of disability from dementia, support for informal caregivers is paramount. Adalsteinn Brown, recent assistant deputy minister at the Health System Strategy Division in Ontario's Ministry of Health and Long-Term Care, has pointed out that health human resources are the most economic, effective, and necessary support systems for Ontario's aged population. If informal caregivers were paid an hourly rate, their bill for Canadian seniors in 2007 would have totaled more than $24 billion. This figure did not include the number of family leave hours taken by caregivers working outside the home. Caregiver burden in Canada is growing: Informal caregiving for Alzheimer's disease requires 231 million hours per year, and this will increase to 756 million hours for the next generation.

8

THINK BEFORE YOU EAT

Among all of the possible self-medications for stress, my vice is comfort food. When I was a child, I was fortunate to be able to eat sweets and junk food and remain skinny. At around age 30, I began to lose my stick-figure shape. At first, the reason was an increase in muscle bulk. I was able to schedule in a lot of athletic training for a while, but later, as I had less flexibility with work hours, I did not expend as much energy. I didn't allow this to keep me from eating just as much as before, however. I was in great cardiovascular condition, but I had a higher body fat content. In fact, what my parents call my "expensive tastes" resulted in a "muffin top." (For those who have somehow escaped this phrase, it refers to the flab above the hipbones that may bulge above the waistband of your pants. The male version is the "spare tire.") I imagine the term "muffin top" is meant to make this part of the body sort of cute and non-threatening, but waist-to-hip measurement ratio (the waist should be smaller than the hip circumference) is an important correlate for health risk. That ratio is more in vogue today than waist circumference alone or body mass index (BMI) as an indicator of health. Is this the return of the "36–24–36" standard?! BMI is equal to body mass (in kilograms) divided by the square of the person's height (in metres). This biases the BMI in favor of the tallest people, since it will take more weight for them to have a higher BMI. The proportion of ideal weight to height differs between sexes and body types. A short, heavy-boned man will appear to have an abnormally high BMI no matter what he does.

Currently, my body fat percentage is an indicator of how much stress I'm under. Stress can lead to overeating if I'm not being mindful about whether I'm truly hungry or just trying to distract myself from stressors. Overeating leads to undesired changes in my shape, which decreases self-esteem, causing my brain to release more cortisol than I want it to when I perceive the next stressor, and the high cortisol-releasing days add up. So it behooves me to address two aspects of the vicious cycle: respond to stress without regressing into comfort-eating wherever possible; and shift my sense of which food items ultimately provide comfort in a sustainable way. At one extreme, the muffin top is an indicator that I am on the precipice above a long downward slope into the Metabolic Syndrome.

One of my colleagues put this terrifying image in my head: Consider that extra belly fat as a satellite source of insulin and hormones produced from fat. We're talking about the hormones that put coarse facial hair on women and droopy breasts on men! I take it one step further and consider that extra body fat to be an alien device that can remotely control my body. The fat releases hormones on its own; it also releases inflammatory factors that have been implicated in the demise of neurons! Keeping this in mind can keep me from reaching for super-tasty potato chips too often.

Metabolic Syndrome, sometimes mysteriously referred to as Metabolic Syndrome X, describes a vicious cycle of obesity and an imbalance of glucose and insulin. Patients with Metabolic Syndrome have high blood pressure, uncontrolled glucose levels, and high lipid (cholesterol) levels that are both caused by the obesity and contributing to it. One usually reads about Metabolic Syndrome in the context of premature death due to heart attack and stroke, but the factors that cause Metabolic Syndrome are also very much related to risk for Alzheimer's disease.

I received a heads-up about this from an anonymous caller to the VA hospital in Los Angeles years ago. I was a Fellow in Behavioral Neurology, and it was a busy clinic day. The caller said he was a community doctor, and he felt very strongly that someone should be looking into the connection between insulin and Alzheimer's disease. I replied that I could see how diabetes and stroke went hand in hand, and that could lead to vascular dementia, which is different from Alzheimer's disease—but he insisted. He had observed casually that many of his diabetic patients seemed to have Alzheimer's disease. As a cocky youngster, I dismissed him by saying I would keep my eyes peeled, meanwhile shaking my head over this "poor generalist" who didn't know the difference between vascular dementia and Alzheimer's disease. I admit that, at the time, I was also unmotivated because I didn't consider myself at risk for diabetes or Metabolic Syndrome.

Approximately four years later, I remembered this conversation and realized how wrong I was when a Columbia University group published its data on how chronically high insulin levels in the blood, not necessarily full-blown diabetes, constitute a risk factor for Alzheimer's disease that has a similar impact across ethnic groups.

Consumption of simple carbohydrates rings alarm bells in the pancreas to release insulin in response. Insulin levels that are too high, like cortisol levels that are too high, set one up for an unhealthy brain in the future.

Cookies have a high glycemic (simple carb) index, but homemade granola can taste as good while delivering a softer glycemic punch. Fruits have glycemic indices that can range too high to be useful. A shot of orange juice is perfect for a diabetic person who has taken her insulin on schedule but has had an unforeseen interruption in her eating schedule. She needs something quickly to prevent a precipitous drop in blood sugar. For most of us, though, a long, tall glass of orange juice could also precipitate the same delayed "sugar-low" observed in a child 30 minutes after eating a sugary breakfast cereal, because a big blast of glucose into the system results in a large secretion of insulin to match it, which produces lethargy. Checking the glycemic indices of commonly consumed foods will reveal that the most unhealthy thing about french fries is that they are made from potatoes, which have a very high glycemic index.

Whole grains can be very good for the body, depending on how they are packaged. Pulverizing whole grains into flour means that the sugars enter the digestive system much more rapidly, rocketing one's blood-glucose level. Eating carbohydrates in the form of whole grain, there is more "low-dose continuous release" action. In working with patients who have diabetes, I already knew that fructose was something to be avoided unless accompanied by fiber that made it harder to absorb and turn into body fat, but I didn't realize that this information holds true for all of us.

The same reasoning explains why it is easier on the body to take in carbohydrates along with some protein. Some of us interpret that liberally as an invitation to have bacon with our toast, but the hard-boiled egg with toast is the better option since it's lower in fat and cholesterol.

Insulin abnormalities like glucose intolerance or insulin resistance create more risk for stroke and vascular dementia than Alzheimer's disease, but they are important alterable factors for both types of dementia. One chapter in the story about how diabetes and insulin are related to Alzheimer's disease entails the abnormally sticky version of protein tau. Whereas there are some connections between insulin and amyloid, insulin resistance caused by a high-fat diet may lead tau into forming the building blocks of neurofibrillary tangles, the other hallmark proteinopathy of Alzheimer's.

In the 1950s, the publications of my grandmother's day didn't even bother writing about indicators of good health. Typical Hawai'ian Island fare included pineapple, abundant sweets, fried foods, and salty foods. Ah Quan sautéed vegetables such as bittermelon with pieces of *lap cheong*, a very fatty sausage considered the Chinese equivalent of kielbasa. When she didn't have *lap cheong* in stock, she'd throw in bacon instead.

My grandparents were people who had survived two world wars and plenty of rationing, so they might not have taken well to elective dietary restrictions. While rationing would have decreased the amount of refined sugar consumed, high-fat foods and the unhealthy forms of carbohydrate were used to fill most bellies. The Depression-era Joads in Steinbeck's *The Grapes of Wrath* are a reminder of how far grease and flour can be stretched in a pinch. Produce was not subject to the same rationing as sugar, flour, and red meat. My mother recalls that the dietary fare at Ah Quan's house always featured moderate proportions of vegetables, before and after World War II. There are indications that this type of diet appears to have a better protective effect for Alzheimer's disease in women than in men.

Diet, therefore, may be an advantage I have over Ah Quan. My anti–muffin top vanity has motivated me to read more about what and how much I can eat while still being a snob about food. The Mediterranean Diet hits a lot of high notes on my checklist for palatable healthy choices. Researchers have replicated findings that this diet—which favors whole grains over processed flour, eating protein more often in the form of fish as opposed to red meat, and enjoying more fruits and vegetables—is not only good for you, but it actually reduces the risk of getting Alzheimer's disease. In fact, half of the dinner plate should have produce on it, with the remaining half split between protein and carbohydrate. I can think of at least two reasons why this set of food choices can work to our advantage: It prevents roller-coasting insulin levels; and it can help reduce body mass index. Hyperglycemia and obesity lead to the development of Metabolic Syndrome.

On the opposite end of the spectrum are those who are too lean. Researchers now believe that low body mass index in late life is correlated with poor cognition. This particular story is still in the chicken vs. egg phase of the telling: Are elders losing weight because their dementing illness is taking away their appetites, or is there something about losing too much body fat that makes one's brain more vulnerable?

Michael Pollan's point in *In Defense of Food* is well taken—beware of food and diet fads! He describes some of the fallacies of popular *orthorexia*, or the obsession with whatever has been deemed The Correct Diet. He correctly points out that a concentration on individual nutrients or components of foods can backfire. When told that it is best to eat less fat, people obeyed, but the price was that they ate a higher proportion of carbohydrates and margarine, and the kicker is that these sacrifices did not decrease calorie consumption.

Ah Quan was advised by her family doctor to increase her intake of omega-3 fatty acids, as found in fish. This advice was implemented as follows: After she cleared her dinner plate (lamb chops, vegetables chopped up with *lap cheong*, and white rice), my grandfather would open up a tin of salmon. She would eat the whole thing, then move on to dessert! If they were out at a restaurant, the tin of salmon was daintily dug out of her handbag and also consumed before dessert. The take-home message is this: Be sure you understand the big picture before you commit to a diet regimen. It is easy for people to get excited and concentrate on one vitamin or supplement, but the human body requires a balance of nutrients in order to sustain good function.

People frequently ask if there are certain vitamins we should take to keep our brains healthy. A widely publicized 1997 study indicated that vitamin E might be good not only for prevention but also for treatment of Alzheimer's disease. However, researchers have been surprised that the results have not been replicated since then.

Biochemists at the time stated that vitamin C should be added if vitamin E were being given as a supplement. My family doctor told me last year that I should be taking vitamin D, and not just because we don't get much sun during the winter. It turns out that the average diet may be deficient in several vitamins, despite the food industry's adding nutrients. I was only taking multivitamins during times when I wasn't eating as many vegetables as I ought to, but I'm going to try to be better about taking them daily. If your liver and kidneys work well, any excess will usually be excreted.

The media—and grocery store shelves—are full of antioxidant claims. My only statement on this is that many foods have antioxidants in them, so we don't have to bore ourselves with daily blueberry binges. The berries may seem more attractive than steamed kale, but all leafy greens are chock-full of the fiber and vitamins we need, in addition to antioxidants.

My father would be glad to know that it was a dentist, Weston Price, who first elucidated that more-natural food, not overly processed or prepared, was better for the body overall. He had been following up on his personal theory that a poor diet was to blame for tooth decay and other dental ailments. There's much more about this in Pollan's book, *In Defense of Food.* Another area of recent debate is toxins. Dr. Joe Schwarcz of the Office for Science and Society at McGill University holds, and I agree, that what makes a substance toxic is often the dose of the substance. Too much of anything can be bad for you. He and his trainees generate articles regularly about any of the latest "scares," which include aluminum and Alzheimer's disease. The information on that subject can be summed up in a sentence: "Please stop worrying about aluminum pots or drinks from aluminum cans." Dr. Joe has also debunked the myth of water filters for me. Most of us in industrialized countries are not gaining anything by putting tap water through charcoal filtration. But we have been taught, through advertising, to expect to be served from a pitcher that filters the water, so it will take a while for that fad to fade out.

Once you know what to eat, then you need to think about how much of it you are eating. It is way too easy to eat protein in excess of your daily required amount. The daily recommended amount of protein—whether fish, fowl, or red meat—is equivalent to the size of your palm. That's not per meal per day; that's the total for the day. I don't know about you, but my palm is much smaller than each of the rib steaks I used to like to eat every week. Bill Cosby jokes, "Did you ever see the customers in health-food stores? They are pale, skinny people who look half dead. In a steak house, you see robust, ruddy people. They're dying, of course, but they look terrific." Whatever protein you consume in excess of what your body needs to build its own proteins is converted to fat. In other words, the muffin top is not made only of muffins. Most laypeople have read enough to automatically envision greasy foods being converted to fat, but even too much protein powder milkshake can lead to obesity.

In addition to watching whether you're overdosing yourself with protein, keep in mind that reducing caloric intake by 33% grants you at least two advantages. (Let's emphasize, this does not apply to those who already are eating small portions adding up to only 1500 kcal per day.) First, the calorie reduction definitely influences BMI, and there are several studies showing that abnormally high BMI is associated with shrinkage of the brain during aging and greater Alzheimer's risk. Allowing BMI to balloon up by four or more points around the time of menopause may have a particularly negative effect on brain volume. Four points could push you from the normal (18.5–24.9) range to overweight (25–29.9), with 30 and over indicating obesity. This gives me incentive to try out the 33% calorie reduction scheme, even if I decide to wait until perimenopause to strictly enforce it.

Second, the 33% calorie restriction benefits the cellular mechanisms referred to as proteostasis. One of the reasons that dementia begins later in life and not in early childhood is that in late life the brain's ability to deactivate and clear its flawed protein products wavers and may be lost. The abnormality in the proteins related to dementia is in the way they are folded, and this origami failure needs to be "tagged and bagged" before it can cause damage to the cell. ("Tag and bag" is an explicit reference to the efficiently morbid approach to clearing dead bodies from a battlefield. Where possible, bodies are identified and labeled accordingly for transport home in bags.) One of the impacts of aging on our cells is that the brain cells' tag-and-bag operations for abnormal protein clearance start to shut down. This process is known more scientifically as the Unfolded Protein Response. When it contributes to an unbalanced ratio between functional, desirable proteins and abnormal ones, clumping of the abnormal protein triggers the downward spiral of neurodegeneration.

If reducing your intake by one-third sounds stressful, understand that that's how you achieve the benefit: The caloric reduction puts enough stress on your cells that the tag-and-bag system is alerted to try harder. This minor stress on the system from being hungry on an internal scale boosts processes that would otherwise slow down because of your advanced age. In brief, one way to counteract age-related slowdowns of cellular waste products is to reduce calories consumed. I like this defense strategy!

Another way to achieve healthy calorie reduction is to minimize mindless eating. There is a mindset—possibly arising from parents who grew up during wartime and experienced deprivation—that we must finish whatever is on our plates. This is dangerous thinking at a time when restaurateurs believe that good value for money is determined by the amount of food on the plate instead of by great taste. Once upon a time, a friend who was refusing to accept what I couldn't finish from my own meal said, "None of us has to be the 'Human Garbage Can.'" Keeping that sentiment in mind could reduce your intake considerably. If you distract yourself with reading (I'm guilty) or television (Guilty!) or email (Guilty!!) while eating, you're distracting yourself from feeling sated. Try *just eating* every once in a while. You may be surprised to find that you've had enough after half as much as you thought you'd need. Consider *not* finishing the serving, but saving it for another seating. With this eating habit, you still get what you had a hankering for, but you don't need to vacuum it all up. Sharing one dessert at the restaurant among the entire table of guests is the way to have *some* cake and eat it too.

Some people will naturally wonder if they can cheat the calorie reduction method for turning on the tag-and-bag system. One lab's creative research explored the effects of calorie reduction in rodents designed genetically to develop a form of Alzheimer's disease. Diet restriction has led to lower amyloid plaque formation (successful tagging and bagging) in those transgenic mice. They followed up on this finding by looking for whatever beneficial compound may be released by the body when calories are reduced by one-third. Resveratrol was that beneficial compound.

The next step was to look for natural sources of resveratrol, to cheat the calorie reduction step. It turns out that resveratrol is in pomegranate juice, as well as the skin of red grapes. This led one lab to create a particular Cabernet Sauvignon wine for its rodents, and the researchers did show that dosing with the lab's "vintage" in lieu of dieting yielded the same positive results as the calorie reduction. For humans, drinking the equivalent amount of wine would lead to medical complications of alcohol intake (cirrhosis, for example). It would not be humanly possible to drink the amount of pomegranate juice necessary, either. So now tens of clinical trials to determine the efficacy of resveratrol supplements are in progress. This demonstrates a robust reticence to surrender our comfort-food habits, which can override considerations for long-term health.

Wine aficionados are happy to note that moderate wine consumption, even after the statistics are adjusted to account for benefits from higher socioeconomic status or access to a more nutritious diet, lowers risk for developing cardiovascular disease and dementia. White wine has been lauded as well as red wine.

The complicating factor is that some of us do not tolerate routine alcohol intake well. This is where genes and culture may determine to what degree an individual can participate in a changeable factor associated with dementia. People genetically programmed toward addiction or depression may exacerbate their conditions if they were to proceed with the wine recommendation, despite avoiding Alzheimer's disease. Another person may meet the disapproval of his community if he is the only imbiber of spirits at the table.

It is worth noting that animal studies do not always predict success or failure in humans. The small differences in species' genomes may make some findings non-transferable. We are, however, most closely related genetically to chimpanzees, fierce omnivores. Comparative neuroscientists like Tuck Finch at the University of Southern California and Robert Sapolsky (see Chapter 7 for a discussion of cortisol) have raised the question of whether the development of proteins to process red meat has also led to our vulnerability to Alzheimer's disease through Apolipoprotein E, since Apolipoprotein E is used in handling the cholesterol we encounter in meat-eating.

The discovery of Creutzfeld–Jakob disease resulting from the consumption of beef raised public consciousness in two ways. People rethought the option of vegetarianism, once they were told that cows were being fed animal matter. We living things are all connected. Furthermore, there was an awakening to some ugly truths about processed foods. Most people find it abhorrent to consider animals being ground up and fed to surviving herdmates. There is an element of cannibalism that we disdain and, in the case of bovine spongiform encephalopathy and Creutzfeldt–Jakob disease, the realization that sick animals were being included as a cattle feed ingredient was too much to bear.

Food is fuel for the body and the brain, but it also has cultural significance and social meaning. In Chinese culture, heaven is a big happy banquet table brimming over with food. Those who go to heaven enjoy eating with six-foot-long chopsticks because each person is feeding the person sitting across from him; hell is the place where everyone is starving because they insist on trying to feed themselves with the same long chopsticks. To Chinese caregivers of patients with dementia, one of the most stressful symptoms of the dementia is loss of appetite and cessation of eating. This loss of quality of life is worse to them than the patient's not being able to live independently or to recognize family members' faces.

Dharma teacher Phillip Moffitt says that everyone has issues with food. It is something we can control about our own bodies, and what we eat, how we eat it, and with whom we eat it is a statement. His compassionate advice is to consider whether your eating preferences are causing suffering, first to you, then to others. Some will choose vegetarianism so as not to cause suffering to the animals; some will choose more healthful foods to consume to prevent Metabolic Syndrome, also known as the "Alien Fat Mass Remotely Controlling My Body." The most significant point from all I have read on this subject is that we owe due diligence to understanding what we are consuming and how it gets onto our plates.

When people ask me about the role of diet for brain health, my answer includes key words about avoiding sugar highs and lows and doing what it takes to keep body fat low. Gaining weight between ages 50 and 55 is most specifically tied to cognitive impairment down the line, so if it's hard for you to control your diet, set your sights on that time period. But start practicing now if you're younger than 50, because old habits die hard!

I must admit I more frequently associate what's on my plate with my muffin top—it is, after all, easier to see what's in the mirror than to see 40 years into the future.

PHYSICAL ACTIVITY AND THE BODY–MIND CONNECTION

Some of my friends admit that they are exercising only so that they can eat. Other friends are using exercise to sculpt their bodies into perfection. It is more than a simple matter of caloric input and calories burned while exercising: People burn calories just by being alive and breathing, and the rate at which an individual can burn calories during rest or during rigorous exercise is related to hormonal balance, whether they are male or female, their age, genetics, and the type of exercise.

Most people have already detected that our caloric metabolism changes over time. I once stepped onto a fancy high-tech weight scale at a health exhibit. The machine coughed out some statistics that sounded like a fortune you'd buy for a quarter on Coney Island: It told me how much of my body consisted of water, gave an estimate of my meat-to-bone ratio, and said I had the metabolism of a 12-year-old. I'd like to believe that was true, but given my already-present muffin top, I'm sure they sell many more scales when the demo machine specs are set to "generous."

A BMI in the low *but not lowest* range is desirable for cardio-vascular longevity, but that package usually comes with low bone density, especially if you're a small-boned woman. So even if you were born under the lucky genetic stars of high metabolism and small body frame, you should do some weight-bearing exercise for the sake of your bones and to maximize tolerance to falls.

Most research on physical fitness and cognitive impairment has focused on delaying or preventing the onset of Alzheimer's disease, and there was a short period when it seemed that the benefits of exercise were enjoyed by women but not necessarily by men. The current state-of-the-art research indicates that both men and women benefit from regular exercise, recently quantified as 150 minutes in total per week. One positive effect of exercise is on blood flow (and therefore oxygen delivery) to the brain from improved cardiovascular tone.

Being part of the San Diego community during my residency years meant assimilation into the Land of the Exercise Freaks. Southern California—and San Diego in particular—is noted as a year-round training haven for triathletes. Attending physicians throughout my residency modeled the balance of hard work inside the hospital and avid recreational exercise outside of it. Judging by their devotion to physical activity, one would think you could get banned from the city if you weren't participating in at least one annual biathlon. The weather and terrain lend themselves to a multitude of opportunities for the active life, whether you like to move vertically or horizontally, through water, over land, or up rocks.

Until that time, exercise had been more of a social activity (a way to meet boys) for me than anything else. But after the long, intense hours at work, the role of exercise in my life transformed into a daily opportunity to let off steam. I converted to a jock lifestyle. Many of us drove trucks or SUVs that we could use as rolling lockers—after work you could make a spur-of-the-moment decision to take advantage of the perfect surfbreak or a pickup game of Ultimate Frisbee. Having chattered my teeth through four Chicago winters, I was more than ready to embrace this new way of life.

My time in San Diego allowed me to build myself into an athlete, and I have been interested to know whether this, like my higher level of education, can counterbalance any risk I have of developing dementia. Persistence has paid off: I used to rank at the bottom on athletic abilities (as measured miserably with the Presidential Fitness program in the United States), but these days, in competitive events I happily finish consistently just above the median for my age group.

As a child, I never excelled at any physical activity, so it generally doesn't bother me to try new sports and accept solid novice status. I'm filled with gratitude just to be standing among the others at the start line with a race number inked onto my limbs whenever I can get back to La Jolla for the annual Roughwater Swim. I am that same child who was afraid of waves and kelp and fish in the water. Somehow I got over myself, and to have learned this new trick feels glorious. And I'm fortunate that my injuries thus far have only created temporary setbacks.

———————

Driving the body more efficiently relates directly to oxygen consumption, and the field of sports physiology has ramped up, triggered in part by the early writings of Ironman-turned-physiologist Dave Scott. We now know that a body that consumes oxygen very efficiently is usually attached to a brain that is fairly resilient to the downsides of aging. Achieving more with less input seems to be an advantage in many bodily functions.

Some brain areas enlarge after increased activity. Studies have shown that mastering a new motor task, like juggling, leads to structural changes in the brain cells. The areas that control your hands and arms and eyes increase in size. We have been scrambling to see if the same effect holds true if you "exercise" the parts of your brain that carry out cognitive functions, such as naming things, or remembering new information, but there have been no obvious brain enlargements from these activities.

How might exercise help to maintain your intelligence or your ability to retain incoming information? The more new skills you attain, the more opportunities there are for cross-referencing information and greasing up neuronal access to that movement or that cognitive strategy. It seems to work in both the physical realm and the higher cognitive one. A recent study done in Shanghai showed that tai chi chuan was beneficial to cognition, similar to the effect of walking quickly for a half hour at a time. Both of these physical activities resulted in an increase in total brain volume after eight months of the program. The study excluded participants who were already practitioners of tai chi chuan, which raised the question of whether simply participating in a non-aerobic exercise that is novel is as good for the brain as rigorous aerobic exercise. There is also evidence in rats that exercise enhances the release of brain-derived neurotrophic factor (BDNF), which is key to inciting brain plasticity (see Chapter 4). BDNF levels remain elevated even during a two-week break from a regular exercise program!

How much exercise is enough? One could get away with vigorous walking for at least 20 minutes a day, three times a week and reduce the risk of dementia by a third. Exercise does not eradicate the risk of developing dementia, but I still have exercise on my list of things to do to counteract any genetic Alzheimer's risk I carry.

Does the benefit of exercise differ based on the BMI that an individual is carrying? I haven't seen any studies that parse out the relative benefits of exercise according to whether you start off with low-low body fat vs. the normal range vs. obese. Instead, I see evidence that having a high BMI (over 25) in mid-life leads to earlier brain volume loss in late life than normal range BMI. Elevated BMI can also contribute negatively to stress hormone risks for dementia. Once we have a better understanding of BMI and Metabolic Syndrome, we might be able to hone the advice we give on when it is most important to start exercising, if it's not already part of your routine, and how long you must keep it up.

In the meantime, planning the ideal exercise program may be as complicated as individual dietary choices. If sports activities are compromising safety, happiness, and health, it's time to consider a change. I gave up underwater hockey and kickboxing, because there was too much bruising in those contact sports for me. Unsustainable! I was in top cardio fitness condition, but when playing underwater hockey I wasn't nimble enough with my swim fins to avoid getting kicked in the head, and I quit shortly after one game during which the team captain noticed I'd stopped moving in the water. He literally threw me out of the pool onto the side where I came to! (Thanks, Cid.) Participation in a sport that gives you "drain blamage" rates re-evaluation.

Boxing is a big bugaboo topic for us neurologists. When you see the torsional trauma given with a good hook or even uppercut to the jaw in slow motion on TV, consider the fact that the boxer's face squishing to one side is just a proxy for the two halves of his (or her!) brain sloshing in opposite directions from each other and sliding over bony aspects of the skull that can act like a cheese grater. I can almost hear the twanging of the connector between those two halves working hard to keep the neuronal networks of the brain intact. Most people do what they can (air bags in the car, avoiding motorcycle rides) to prevent this type of head trauma, but boxers take it on as a repetitive occupational hazard. The boxer with the glass jaw (one who is easily knocked out with only one blow) may not win, but the glass jaw protects him or her from repetitive blows and marathon rounds, and therefore decreases the risk of chronic traumatic encephalopathy or dementia. Contact sports are a very tough way to make a living.

I've also experienced firsthand, through muay thai kickboxing, what a different type of contact sport this is. Rene Denfeld's *Kill the Body, the Head Will Fall* explains well how boxing creates an outlet for the physical aggression all of us harbor. It also describes the intimacy and trust built into the relationship boxers have with their sparring partners, and how this sport can address the fear of getting hurt. Boxing is an opportunity to learn a lot more about how the body can rise to challenges. But I wish it were easier on the brain.

In a bold, well-timed move, the National Football League is now seriously investigating the fates of players after suffering head trauma. The National Hockey League Alumni Association, led by its current executive director, former Montreal Canadien Mark Napier, has teamed up with my home institution, Baycrest, to follow these athletes for chronic cognitive impairment as they age.

A concern more pertinent to the general population is a single incident of head trauma, especially.

It's worse if this happens before age 18. Your risk of developing Alzheimer's is nearly doubled if you suffered a significant smack to the head in childhood. If you have a first-degree relative with Alzheimer's disease, that already tripled the risk, and the head trauma would bring you up to $2 \times 3 = 6$ times the risk. But it is not clear to me yet at what advanced age the doubling applies. The contribution of childhood traumatic brain injury is a bit counterintuitive, because the two events are so separated by time, but lifespan studies show this greater influence of timing in youth than in either mid- or late life.

Certain activities may yield more of a social benefit for some people than a physiological one. Going for a brisk walk is not without its dangers (watch out for cars and uneven ground!), but it's something you can easily recruit friends to. Right now, we don't know whether the social or the physiological benefit of exercise is more beneficial to the brain in the long run, but I repeat that if an exercise plan allows enjoyment, provides a sense of well-being, and doesn't impinge on safety, it's an important part of a lifelong regimen. Physical activity has shown more robust effects on keeping people's cognition intact than have any medication trials thus far!

The benefits of regular exercise for the brain are adding up all the time. Exercise:

- keeps your BMI low
- reduces stroke risk and possibly eradicates that dementia risk factor
- reduces stress (provided you pick the right activities for your body and personality)
- racks up plasticity points through learning new skills
- creates a social outlet to decrease times of loneliness, which is itself a risk for Alzheimer's disease (see Chapter 10, "Social Networks")
- potentially reduces the risk of falling, which figures large in quality of life and mortality for the elderly; falling and breaking a hip leads to major immobility and therefore is a huge mortality risk factor for an elderly person

There have been unequivocal findings in favor of maintaining as physically active a lifestyle as possible from childhood to old age. Studies of frail elders not only correlate frailty to enhanced morbidity with dementia and hastened mortality, but also show the impact of nutrition, physical activities, leisure activities, and health-related behaviors (engagement with others, regular screening at the doctor's office, compliance with medications) on the severity of any frailty. But exercise training can be done creatively for those who are frail. Dr. Louis Bherer at the University of Quebec at Montreal (UQAM) is showing that exercise tailored to frail older adults can bear cognitive benefits and enhance quality of life.

It may never be too late to start exercising. Evidence dating back to 2010 shows that rigorous exercise supervised by a personal trainer for 45 minutes three times a week enhances attention and mental task-juggling for patients with amnestic mild cognitive impairment, which represent in many cases an early stage of Alzheimer's disease. Patients with dementia can and should remain physically active in sports they had previously mastered. They may not be as accurate in keeping score as before, but if the dementia has not carved away their motivation to pursue the activity, it can bring all the same benefits as before. There has even been an indication in mouse models that exercise helps to clear more amyloid build-up in the brain than does changing from a high- to a low-fat diet, suggesting that maybe it is okay to think about exercising to support one's eating habits! But do both if you can.

10

SOCIAL NETWORKS

By definition, dementia renders a patient dependent upon others for assistance. This accounts for some amount of the fear about dementia. But we are connected to others and rely upon their contributions to our health and productivity on a daily basis. Colleagues, family, and friends are some obvious examples, but there are countless other connections that are often taken for granted, such as how food gets to your table, navigating to your destination by car without incident, and random kindnesses that brighten your day. In a sense, the assistance you might require as a patient with dementia is just another version of the interconnectedness of human life.

If someone has been the pillar of strength for others, consider that the competent person who has taken care of everyone else throughout life may finally experience receiving care when she or he has dementia. The void left by the leader of the family may inspire other family members to gain new confidence in managing the household or to help each other.

When Dorothy, a successful former CEO with a confident smile, came into the Memory Clinic, she was so impeccably dressed, groomed, and warm in greeting that it was hard not to mistake her for a caregiver accompanying a patient. However, she was the patient, and the person who brought her to the clinic was the daughter of a close friend who had become concerned about Dorothy's ability to function on her own. Over the course of four years, Dorothy had descended from being very high functioning and independent to showing strong paranoia, terrible memory loss, and confusion. She had lived alone for decades in a condominium where she had some girlfriends as neighbors; her long-term psychotherapist had an office across the street, and there was a pharmacy in her building. Despite the potential sources of assistance nearby, Dorothy was resistant to help. She was frightened of what the future might hold, and did not want to leave her condo to become an isolated denizen of an assisted-living facility, "or worse yet, a nursing home."

I imagined that she had prided herself and built her ego on her independence, and this latest development ran unfathomably counter to her worldview and sense of place. The internal conflict was so awful that her daily activities had become restricted to dropping in at the pharmacy to see if she could refill her sleeping pills and refusing her psychotherapist's pleas to allow others to help. I think the psychotherapist had been her one confidant for decades.

Her friend's daughter, who held power of attorney, met with my nurse to strategize about the best way to bring needed resources to Dorothy's doorstep. We concentrated on four goals:

to make Dorothy feel safe, healthy, valued, and able to experience joy.

At times like this, I find it easier to hold an open-ended conversation, in which I ask the patient how he or she is feeling, or if there are any requests of the doctor's office. I seldom need to challenge the patient by saying that everyone else feels anxious about her living arrangements. Improvisation is an important skill to bring to the conversation, if the patient wants to distract me from any discussion of dementia or cognitive problems. One helpful question is whether the patient feels safe at home. This may elicit a delusion that someone is stealing from them, or that the patient cannot recognize a visitor who should be familiar.

Sometimes I might ask, "What did you do this weekend?," which can reveal whether the patient is able to enjoy it, to what extent she can remember the story well enough to relate it to me, or if memory fails, confabulation will take over and corroborate the caregiver's account of a disorganized, chaotic life outside of the clinic.

Often, even if the patient cannot do well on memory testing, she is still in good physical shape, and I can concentrate my comments on the positive aspects of the physical exam. At that clinic visit, Dorothy was able to cover for her memory problem by giving some pat, superficial answers. After examining her, I told her she was as strong as a horse and looking great, as always. Dorothy's face brightened into a genuine smile and she thanked me by saying, "You don't know how much that means to me. I just wanted someone to tell me, 'You're doin' okay, Cookie!'" This was qualitatively different from needing a pill to cure the illness. This was a short-term request, purely about how today was going.

Dorothy was so grateful for the benign report card that she said if she weren't worried about me being such a professional, she would give me a hug. I told her I had gotten over that a long time ago and would gladly take the hug. I couldn't help but flash forward in my own mind to the cautionary tale before me: Get used to relying on other people. We are all connected, and there will be times when we need others to help us. There's no time like the present to learn how to let your friends know if you need help. Had she been too professional for hugs?

A United Kingdom research translation group called Foresight reports that well-being arises from five behaviors: (1) Connect; (2) Be active; (3) Take notice; (4) Keep learning; and (5) Give. "Seeing yourself, and your happiness, linked to the wider community can be rewarding and creates connections with the people around you," the report advises.

Social networking is something that might be hard to start late in life. Aspects of our personalities (some genetically determined), culture, geography, occupation, and social circumstances weigh on the degree to which we integrate with others. Meaningful interactions with others are specifically good for the brain. Ah Quan exemplified a life fully plugged into social networks from the very beginning.

My grandfather was a handsome young letter carrier for the U.S. postal service, who was in the newspapers after his horse-drawn mail carriage was struck by one of the first automobiles in Honolulu. He found Ah Quan through her particular girlhood hobby: She cultivated long-term international correspondence with pen-pals. What postman would not be intrigued to meet the Chinese girl, and not someone transplanted from the U.S. mainland, who was receiving such exotic mail? They met at the mailbox in front of the missionaries' house on Judd Street, and he was smitten. At 14, she was considered underage by the Green family and was only allowed to see this 21-year-old letter carrier at the mailbox on delivery days.

The only story Grandma ever told me about life at the missionaries' house was that she had to hide a large box of *toong mai*, a gift from my grandfather. For those unfamiliar with this Chinese sweet, think of gingery Rice Krispie treats with peanuts embedded in them. She solved the problem by crunching and munching her way through the entire box during the wee hours the same night he'd delivered them!

The courtship went on for as long as it took her to graduate from high school (that's a lot of days at the mailbox) and stretched to a total of seven years before they were married. A woman of Ah Quan's generation was much better off if "She had her a man!" This quote comes from Jeanine, a dance classmate whose mother has vascular dementia, when she describes her mother's main concerns through life. "Having a Man" meant financial security, a place to live, a family, and a clear-cut role in all of those parts of life.

These days a woman often needs a job, and I am amused when I hear 10-year-old girls planning their careers. Ah Quan's first job after graduating from high school was as a secretary to the principal, but the job description included teaching sewing on Fridays and recording kindergarteners' growth curves. She was 19 years old at the time, and she made $80 per week (less than $2 an hour). She left the job after almost two years to work as a secretary at the Salvation Army. After three years there, she spent 12 years at home raising my uncle and mother. Her next job was not until 1942, when she became a clerk in the Office of Civilian Defense (eight months after the bombing of Pearl Harbor). This was an interesting job description: She kept records for the medical director, prepared dressings for wounds, and issued liquor and gas coupons. At that point, she was making $150 per week. She was then a secretary at the Humane Society, where she worked for nine years and whence came my mother's family dog, Kuni. Kuni, a black cocker spaniel, got his name from the Cantonese words for "Happy New Year," which are *Kung Hee Fat Choy* and sounds like "Coonie Fott Choy."

At 43, Ah Quan had raised her two children, and they were headed to opportunities on the mainland that didn't yet exist in the Islands. At age 49, Ah Quan applied for a position as a Level I administrative secretary with the City and County of Honolulu Department of Civil Service. She had been working as a temporary administrative secretary at the mayor's office, and people there must have encouraged her to apply to take the position permanently. Ah Quan was working 48-hour weeks at a secretarial desk at the Board of Water Supply: I see that her newsletter column was infused with comments about family life and neighbors. Work was just another part of her life and not the main focus.

Ah Quan was remarkable in that she enjoyed putting special touches on every act, for every person in her life. There were handmade tags to accompany the scarf she'd knitted for the neighbor's kid, the first in the family to go to college on the Mainland; the tin of individually wrapped cookies baked from scratch; and to celebrate a birthday, the lei made from steph-anotis alternating with green roses, all from her garden. This was loving kindness offered to all. Her last words to me were, "Be kind to each other." When she retired, she was just as busy as ever, if not more, interacting with so many friends and relatives. I contrast this against what I see more commonly in the population, where households can be quite insular.

In today's parlance, Ah Quan was a practitioner of mindfulness. It can be difficult to slow down to bring meaning to all social activities in the midst of our fast-paced, multitasking modes. That Ah Quan was bright and talented gave her a wider scope of influence and skills to care for others. I believe her example shaped my approach to my community, to feel most fulfilled when "plugged in" as opposed to keeping to myself.

One of her retirement goals was to extend her 45 years of international pen-pal communications to 50. She had more than exceeded this before she died, and all before Facebook. She had hit all five of the Foresight checklist items for well-being, even if she hadn't scored very high by Nun Study standards.

Social networking, while good for the brain because of the constant novelty and stimulation, may also solidify a safety net for getting support when it's needed. There are no guarantees about what family will do in the tragic event of dementia. I have seen many caregivers who continue their devotion to the patient, but there are healthy families that fall apart under the duress of dementia, and dysfunctional families that become more dysfunctional.

Most studies agree that having a life partner creates an advantage for mortality and morbidity over being single. I don't think it's been decided conclusively that this has only been an advantage for men. People living with a partner in mid-life (having a mean age of 50.4 years) are less likely to show cognitive impairment later in life. If someone is persistently single from mid-life into late life, the risk for Alzheimer's disease is tripled. Depression related to losing a spouse has an even greater impact: widowed people have 7.67 times the risk for Alzheimer's disease that non-widowed people have. Relationships are important. And interestingly, from a social networks point of view, *not* having children can bear an advantage over having children with whom there are stressful or dissatisfying interactions.

We also have to extend ourselves beyond one primary relationship. The idea is that a diversified social portfolio can provide support better than a single social connection. I like a theme that encourages us to reach out to others. Spreading one's efforts to connect can take the pressure off of a single family member or friend. Counting on an adult child as a primary caregiver may not be fair to the child and may reduce incentive to interact meaningfully with peers and other community members in a mutually supportive network.

One striking example of this was a Chinese-speaking woman transferred from another hospital to our inpatient unit for behaviorally disturbed patients. Mrs. Tang was from a rural area in the People's Republic of China and had been brought to Toronto after her sons had settled into new lives with their spouses and children. The transfer notes from the original facility diagnosed her as having a dementia that had started fairly recently. Upon her arrival, one of my colleagues clued me in to the possibility that this woman might have been misdiagnosed due to a language barrier and the absence of a full history of her symptoms.

Her family members were difficult for the hospital staff to reach. Her son was busy working two jobs. Her grandson, who spoke English well, had not spent much time with his grandmother and could not answer questions about how she had been functioning one year ago, two years ago, or even two weeks ago. The son with two jobs told a staff person through a translator that he could make himself available once a week, but this was not intended to be a visit to his mother. The grandson seemed to be the only one who would come and spend a little time with her, but they did not seem to converse or discuss her needs.

When I walked into her room to introduce myself in broken Mandarin, I found a woman who did not seem that old, only in her early sixties, lying on her back in bed with the back of her hand against her forehead in a pose as if she were languishing, eyes closed. Despite my mispronunciation, her eyes popped open at my greeting, and she immediately began speaking to me as if she had found a new friend. I was embarrassed and sorry that I could neither understand nor answer her questions in Mandarin. When I stated my well-practiced "I hear you but I do not understand you," Mrs. Tang's eyes dulled and she turned away from me in what I imagined was disgust. This corroborated what my colleague had reported, and it was distressing to learn that at that time we had no translators easily available at our hospital.

The next morning, Mrs. Tang was wandering the halls of the locked unit, seemingly bored out of her skull, dragging her feet and watching everything through half-open eyes. A cantankerous, volatile neighboring patient provided the only excitement of the day, but this was frightening and upsetting. The next-door neighbor would, on a very rapid cycle, cuddle a stuffed black-and-white cow, then suddenly spout out expletives and throw the cow to the ground. I was standing right there when she threw the cow at Mrs. Tang. Who would not have thrown it right back at her? Mrs. Tang's day consisted of hours of absolute boredom interrupted by moments of sheer terror. To be abandoned at a hospital, isolated by language and a shaky diagnosis, was a terrible situation. I doubt that her family intended for her to feel abandoned, and this was one of the most awful examples of how having children would not necessarily guarantee caregiver support for one's darkest cognitive or behavioral moments.

How could we help this woman to feel safe and understood, or add some brightness to her day? The circumstances of her immigration had disconnected her from her lifelong, familiar social network. When I walked back from the hospital unit to my clinic on the other side of the facility, I recalled that Mindy had traveled through China recently. I asked her if she had printed any of the photos that were taken along the way. Timing is everything. It just so happens that Mindy's husband had printed duplicate copies of all their photos, because this family likes to organize hard copy photo album keepsakes. She gladly donated many photos. The unit staff quickly compiled these into a photo album for Mrs. Tang, and it made all the difference. She kept it very close to her for the rest of her stay. From the inpatient unit, Mrs. Tang went to a nursing home, where I am hoping she has been able to gain some sense of community.

Isolation correlates with a higher risk of dementia. Lou Cozolino, a psychology professor at Pepperdine University, has pointed out that single-family households can create silos of isolation, whereas the traditional concept of a tribal community incorporates members of all ages and abilities within its network of interdependence. Cozolino has described how his work as a psychotherapist taught him that the healing process entails re-incorporation of elders into the community.

When I was researching the cultural differences keeping people from seeking medical attention for dementia, I was reminded that in Asian cultures, as opposed to Caucasian North American, older people are kept very active within the mainstream community. This builds upon research that champions engagement of the mind for improved brain aging. Instead of being relegated to seniors' residences, each family's elders in the old Asian tradition stay within the multigenerational household, fulfilling roles as cook, housekeeper, gardener, or babysitter. While not expected to contribute to the household income, they have obligations to fulfill, and the job description has a sliding scale, according to level of ability.

Sometimes I wonder if I'm one of those very people I try to avoid sitting next to on airplanes, the overly chatty who are unable to let the traveler sleep or have treasured quiet time for reading. I don't talk to everyone, but I sometimes strike it rich, in terms of finding someone with whom there is a serendipitous shared interest. On a flight to Vancouver, I noticed that my seatmate had brought a manuscript for the five-hour plane ride, just like I had. She was Arlene Katz, a social medicine expert, and she had formed a Council of Elders to help teach family-medicine trainees at Harvard how *successfully* aging people live and problem solve. This type of information is missing from the medical school curriculum. The fledgling doctors in Arlene's program bring their difficult cases before the Council and value what they are told, gaining the kind of wisdom that doesn't come from a book. This is a terrific new teaching resource, aimed at weaving otherwise disenfranchised elders back into the community in a meaningful way, not as impaired persons.

Paul Baltes, a lifespan psychologist at the Max Planck Institute in Berlin, did not live to complete his book about wisdom, entitled *Wisdom as Orchestration of Mind and Virtue*, but many have taken encouragement about aging from his manuscript. While advancing age may be accompanied by physical ailments, the experiences over a long lifetime grant wisdom that shows a coordination of cognition, motivation, and emotion; the ability to prioritize values and see things in context; the ability to advise and manage others (not just self); recognition and management of uncertainty (not just tolerance of it); and spiritual reflection.

Another way for older adults and youth to interact in ways that are beneficial to both is through intergenerational school programs. Patients with dementia participate as volunteers to read to kindergarten classes or to share life history reminiscences with older children, allowing them to contribute and to join in the excitement of a young person's learning. The students benefit from having someone teach from real-life experience. Whether through a council of elders or volunteer work, the elderly, even with cognitive impairment, can and should remain integrated with the community.

Unfortunately, some symptoms of dementia can preclude a leadership role and instead require supervision for safety. Many of my patients with frontotemporal dementia are too young to fit in at day programs designed for those with Alzheimer's disease. However, the 20-year age gap between participants can, in some cases, be bridged by giving the younger patient the impression that she or he is at the day program as a volunteer to help the others. One day program in Toronto even prints out "paychecks" to distribute biweekly to these participants. This is a terrific example of allowing someone to feel like he's an active contributor to a community that will embrace him as he is.

One day when several of us were catching up on news of patients who had passed away during the week, I was caught by surprise that a patient I had seen only six weeks previously was on that deceased list. Before I had time to process why this news saddened me so much, someone at the conference room table, noting my change of expression, suggested facetiously, "Do you think Adie's husband killed her?" That heightened the sense of distress that I had felt on the first and only day that I had met Adie. This woman and her husband had reached their nineties. She had seemed grossly impaired in cognition, but once we outfitted her with an amplifier to compensate for her hearing loss, we found that she was not as deeply into Alzheimer's disease as she had seemed.

I was delighted to find that once she could hear, she was able to demonstrate a strong and humorous personality. This was a woman with spunk! But the visit took us on an emotional roller-coaster, because once we had settled upon the likely diagnosis and a treatment plan, her husband, who was approximately four years her senior, refused on the spot to supervise her medications or take her to a physiotherapist to address the disabled shoulder that we had discovered on neurological examination.

I know that couples who have been together as long as they have often figure out a workable distance at which to coexist, but I had hoped that understanding her condition would have recruited him to be more of a caregiver. When we inquired about whether there were any close friends or children who might be able to step in to help, her husband told us that they had a son who lived in town, but he was not to be bothered.

The night of that first visit, I couldn't help but think of that case once I'd returned to my singleton household. It underscored the point that there are no guarantees about who will be willing to provide care. That Adie died so unexpectedly was somehow not as saddening as the declaration of isolation I had heard at that first appointment.

Evidence from research about social networks reveals that interacting with your community is important when it comes to maintaining brain health. Community is not only genetically defined. Children can be one aspect of a support system, but there are many other possible links to others who can help; colleagues, neighbors, and friends are important too. In the case of neurobiologist Robert Sapolsky's baboons, even the alpha male must create connections with other members of the troupe. There will come a day when he is no longer the dominant figure, due to injury and aging, and those baboons that he has taken time to groom will later share food with him or protect him from younger, competitive males. The impact of isolating oneself from company is powerful.

11

TREATMENT BEGINS
WITH THE DOCTOR–PATIENT
RELATIONSHIP

How can any of us fight an uphill battle against an illness currently without cure? To defer to a higher power day in and day out is not every physician's cup of tea. I chose dementia as my focus because in ways that I recognized early on, and in others that I discovered later, this type of clinical work and research allows me to bring my philosophy on life into daily practice. I'm constantly challenged to develop my skills, which don't automatically arise from good intentions. While I hope my colleagues and I are following the right paths to curing dementia and treating our patients, there is even more to do for the family living with a confused elder today. The reconciliation between working for a better future and facilitating a better today involves skills I did not learn in medical school.

Dementia has touched so many people's lives. Since leaving Los Angeles, I return at Christmastime to visit family and attend my old ballet class. The last time I had coffee with some of the women after class, it turned out that the teacher's father was affected by Alzheimer's disease, and a classmate's mother had

156

vascular dementia. Experience has taught me that the key to not becoming overwhelmed by the sheer number of these sad stories is not to listen as someone who is expected to fix the problem. Instead, just listen. This runs counter to the justifications that we listed for being chosen on our medical school applications. The intention to help is strong, but the skillful execution of that intent is to scale the energy output to the need.

In fact, I have found that trying to meet each medical complaint with a proposed solution can achieve the opposite effect of helping: I can upset both the caregiver and myself! Case in point: Caregiver Betty says that nothing I suggest will work, but she hasn't tried any of it and doesn't want to. To a certain extent, I dread this type of visit. Typically it takes me 10 minutes of this exasperating back-and-forth to realize that she doesn't want me to fix any of the problems she's reporting. Betty needs for me to *hear* what she's going through as a caregiver to someone with a dementia that neither of them wished for, full stop.

A colleague once arranged for me to dine with an astronaut friend of his while I was away at a conference. Who wouldn't jump at such a chance? I was greeted by an older man who fit the profile; he was lean, distinguished, and Spartan. But David seemed to be looking down his nose at me. Given what he had achieved in life, I decided it was within his rights to do so and carried on with the evening, figuring I would at least learn something new. Halfway through the walk from our meeting place to the restaurant, he stopped in the road and grumbled, "You know, I had to think twice about agreeing to dinner with a neurologist when I obviously have a movement disorder!!" I will admit that, when waiting at an airport or other public places, my mind will make instant diagnoses, but when I'm enjoying the sights and sounds of a new city, doctor-mode does not click on so automatically.

I replied, "I had noticed something about your eyes," but left him to decide if we would talk about it. Some part of me was curious; another part of me did not want to work during a long, beautiful sunset. But this open invitation prompted David to unload about frustrating medication trials for what his doctors had called blepharospasm, an involuntary squeezing shut of the eyes. The fact that I had not at all recognized his signs as blepharospasm made silence very easy for me. Not only did David have a lot to get off his chest, but I didn't have the skills to interrupt him with counteradvice. He had tried three different medications, and one of them had led to horrible feelings of depression and even suicidal thoughts. It doesn't take a medical education to be able to empathize with that and to express relief that the person has stopped taking that medication. We stood there in the road until he had gotten the entire story out of his system, then we continued walking—in retrospect, I'd like to say that it was with a lighter step.

Over dinner, I learned how rigorous the testing for an astronaut can be. It is right out of the movie *The Right Stuff*, but much less glamorous. For someone like me, who is claustrophobic, some of the procedures he described would constitute inhumane torture. Imagine being zipped up inside a beanbag chair, with nothing else inside but the darkness; there are no extra holes for air, and the test supervisors neglected to mention how long the test will be run. As someone who had aspired all his life to be an astronaut, he probably had the foresight to visit the bathroom before reporting for any tests. David handled the situation much better than I would have. He explained that early in life he'd developed the ability to detach his mind from the rest of his body, and this skill allowed him to simply take a nap once they closed the beanbag around him. The dinner conversation was, as expected, very interesting and thought-provoking. When David walked me back to my hotel, he thanked me for having listened to his neurological tale, and we parted ways.

I woke up early the next morning with a hunch about David's "blepharospasm." The beanbag chair was only one anecdote he'd related over dinner. Something in his childhood had incited the need for mental dissociation. The reason I had not jumped to the conclusion of blepharospasm when we first met is that, instead of being squinched tightly closed, David's eyelids were drooping loosely over his eyes, forcing him to tilt his head back and literally look down his nose to be able to see anything. No wonder the medications for blepharospasm had not worked! But what would?

I called David to propose an intervention. I asked him to wear a pair of sunglasses to meet me at a public park bench. I also wore sunglasses as I explained what I had in mind. Since he had hinted the previous evening at some significant events from his childhood that allowed him to become perfect for astronaut work, I told him I thought the same strength might be causing his current problem. He was mentally shutting himself off from the external world for too long, and perhaps his body was overcompensating by physically shutting his eyes to what was happening around him. I admitted it was a hokey, armchair-psychologist approach, and I made disclaimers about not having completed a psychiatric residency. But I told him I was open to hearing his story, and our sunglasses were to assist us in just getting the words out, without reacting to them or to each other.

Sometimes people encountered while traveling make terrific confidants because they don't know the other characters in the story, they likely will never meet them, and they can listen more objectively than our close friends. This was one of those times. David told me about inappropriate sexual advances from his mother, which he kept secret as a boy in hopes that he was sparing his brothers the same abuse. Similar unwanted sexual attention came from staff at a hospital where he had volunteered as an adolescent. When he reported this to his father, his father refused to believe it, did not support his son, and expected him to continue working there. David had suffered yet another betrayal of his personal space. This explained perfectly why he was so talented at dissociating mind from body. Without this skill, he would never have survived and succeeded in his chosen profession.

I didn't say anything until David was completely done with his story. I didn't have to. Of course I wondered if his eyes would open up, but in keeping with the theme of freeing him from having to perform for me, I did not ask him to take his sunglasses off. We wrapped up the meeting with him saying he felt better and thanking me for my time. He said he wanted to show me something, took off his sunglasses, and showed me his two eyes, wide open. Even more gratifying was when he emailed me the next day to report that his dinner date that night had remarked that she had never noticed how beautiful his eyes were. This disabling eye-shutting had caused him to get into bicycle accidents, and apparently the condition was

TREATMENT BEGINS WITH THE DOCTOR–PATIENT RELATIONSHIP

more responsive to someone compassionately listening than it had been to medication. This is a neuropsychiatric case, one in which the mind–body connection is strong and it's not clear whether the nerve-to-motor short circuit or the psychological conflict occurred first.

My family frequently quotes a hilarious line from Jay Ward's cartoon, "Dudley Do-Right of the Mounties." The context is that the commissioner's daughter is yet again tied to the railroad tracks. In a sentence form of spoonerism, the panicked commissioner commands Dudley, "Don't just do something, stand there!" Sometimes a patient's family doesn't want me to problem solve; that is a distraction from compassionately acknowledging their situation, which Betty's friends and other family members may not be able to do, for reasons of their own. Stillness can bring kindness and peace to those nearby.

Sometimes we can't just listen, out of aversion to tragedy. Aversion makes us want to turn away from the painful story. Some people who cannot listen with compassion are often reminded, "It's not all about *you*!!" This is an important point for physicians to remind ourselves, because the way the medical system is structured does revolve around us, especially in Canada where there is a doctor shortage. It does look like it's all about us. The patient waits for an appointment to see us. We went through a lot of training to be repositories for knowledge, and patients come to us with questions. It's easy to romanticize the scenario into families climbing the mountain to reach us and hear our wisdom at the summit. It runs counter to most physicians' worldviews to admit that they don't have a cure or better news. It does feel very uncomfortable to be the bearer of bad news on the day we confirm a diagnosis of Alzheimer's disease. If we consider ourselves to be hosts and patients have trekked all the way up the mountain to visit, the least we could do would be to serve up some tea and read out an auspicious fortune. But the doctor–patient relationship is not about bolstering the physician's ego.

Some would abbreviate the tenets of Buddhism with an aphorism, "No self, no problem." This reminds us that we are all connected, that there is no one person who will always be the hub of activity and purpose, and that since everything changes, we can always strive to detach ourselves from thoughts of self-importance or victimization or pride. Telling a person he has a progressive dementia is a job that someone has to do, hopefully with the right amount of compassion and kindness for the circumstances. The other alternative is to send patients away under- or misinformed.

During the summer between my first and second years of medical school, my master's degree work in marine biology earned me an Alaskan sea adventure. The small marine biology department at Sheldon Jackson College needed help creating teaching videos on the microhabitats in the waters surrounding Sitka, Alaska. I had full access to the holdings of the college library. My summer job there was to wake up in time to catch the boat to spectacular sites and capture video content. We were not salaried but were housed in the summer Elderhostel. I've never dined so consistently on fresh seafood in my life.

The art and totem poles of the Haida and Tlingit spoke to

me as soon as I saw them in Sitka. I come from Los Angeles, where people regularly speak of having been someone or somewhere "in a previous life." I can't say that I imagined myself to be a Northwest First Nations elder in a previous life, but I will say that this was one of the places where I felt a compelling resonance, a sense of belonging to something much larger and enduring. This type of perspective is very helpful when we need to be reminded that we cannot control the day-to-day events in our lives, and that the overall flow over time is more important.

In one gorgeous explanation of how a Haida shaman would diagnose a villager's problems, the shaman would paddle her canoe out to the kelp forest, in preparation for a swim to the sea bottom. Once at the bottom, she would request a visit with the Sea-Witch, whose hair, like the longest strands of kelp extending to the ocean's surface, was invariably tangled. The shaman would soothe the Sea-Witch by combing and untangling this impossible hair, and the Sea-Witch, lulled into cooperation, would divulge the reason and cure for the ailment up on land. The lesson was that helping others would require thoughtful observation, journeys of discovery, and an ability to brave unpleasant or downright frightful situations. In a medical context, this can translate to working through the aversive reaction in order to make oneself fully present and available to someone in need.

On one medical school rotation, I spent a lot of time with an old Italian patient, Aldo, who had a diagnosis of BOOP. BOOP stands for Bronchiolitis Obliterans Organizing Pneumonia, which requires heavy steroid treatment to keep the body's immune response from shutting off oxygen delivery into the body. At his worst, Aldo was suffocating right before our very eyes. Being on-call overnight as a medical student allows us time to sit with our patients, time that isn't granted again later in training when we have responsibility for more people or as our evenings are taken up by grant applications. But at age 24, I sat on the edge of Aldo's bed one night after he'd finished dinner. Aldo had tubes for oxygen lightly placed in his nostrils, but while we were talking, I was watching the monitor on his finger. When it dropped too low, he had to switch to a clear plastic mask that fit over his nose and mouth to deliver oxygen to his body more effectively. In my selfish way, I didn't want him to die on my watch! His coughing fits were terrifying, causing the monitor to peal alarms.

I distracted myself (and maybe him) from this awful coughing by asking who was in the photo frame on his night-stand. Only patients who know they'll be hospitalized for a long haul bring these types of personal effects to their rooms. This prompted him to spend an hour telling me about how much he loved his wife, was proud of his children, and missed his little dog Freeway terribly during the long hospitalization. I listened. I realized how privileged I was to sit with this tough guy with tears leaking from his eyes. I thanked him for telling me, and the next day, I went on to the next medical student rotation. He seemed stable, so I looked forward to dropping by to say hello informally the following week.

But when I returned to his room, he was gone, and the resident who had been caring for him told me Aldo had died. My eyes teared up and my throat closed, but I wasn't sure if it was "okay" for me to have felt so emotionally attached to one of my patients. We had been schooled that if we can't maintain objectivity, we may not be able to serve our patients as well. "*Do you*

KNOW what equanimitas *means*?"—the question I'd been asked long ago came back to me. I felt a little ashamed at my emotional response to the news and hastily excused myself before I could be "voted off the island" of doctorhood.

How can a person not feel bonded to someone who shares such intimate things? I wrote to his family, transcribing all I could remember from my last conversation with Aldo. His wife and I corresponded every Christmas for almost 20 years afterward. Freeway lived a very long time, and Aldo's wife felt the dog still looked for his master. I did not cure Aldo, and I did not prolong his life, but I was able to address his anxiety about imminent death and to acknowledge his family's suffering.

Feeling uncomfortable about mourning the loss of Aldo raised my first conflict over where exactly the doctor–patient relationship's boundaries lie. If caring about patients motivates the study of medicine, how do students avoid getting "too attached"? Exactly how attached is "too attached"? Certainly, having favorite patients who get much more attention than others is a clear no-no. And becoming incapacitated by grief if a patient dies is simply dysfunctional. But what if a patient extends an invitation to join the family for dinner? Is that okay—is it rude to refuse?

One of my patients with a drastic change in language function was coming to clinic appointments by himself. Most of my patients arrive accompanied by a spouse or adult child. This is because they have lost their driving privileges due to their diagnosis of dementia, or family members do not count on them to remember what the doctor said to do after the appointment.

In Leonard's case, it was not clear to me whether his wife did not realize he had a serious, progressive illness, or whether she did not care. When I first asked after her, Leonard had told me that she was busy and had other things to do. While his language problem kept him from reciting her phone number to me, it was not interfering with his ability to drive a car safely at the time, and so he could come to appointments by himself.

After a year of his language's continuing to decline, though, I thought it would be good to meet her so that we could talk together about Leonard's future needs. When I finally did meet Judie, I recognized her as a kindred spirit immediately, and she invited me to join them for dinner. This set off all kinds of alarms, mostly about maintaining a safe distance, about maintaining "equanimity." If I got too attached, would I be allowing emotions to rule? I decided that as adults, we could deal with requests for inappropriate favors if and when they came up. And I didn't have to protect myself from getting too attached to someone whom I would soon lose. I wasn't sure if the illness would lead to a premature death for Leonard; he was already well into his seventies and might die from something more typical, like a heart attack, as opposed to the illness I was treating him for.

When we finally sat down together at the dinner table, I confided to Judie my misgivings about maintaining a professional doctor–patient relationship. She laughed at me, saying she would cure me of that. We have been close friends ever since, and in many instances I have called her my Fairy Godmother. She calls me, "Saint Tiffany," which of course always brings me crashing right down to earth where I belong.

Later, while I was on a ski trip in Colorado, one of my former neurology professors interrupted the vacation with a phone call to request that I see his old friends as soon as I returned to L.A. I was flattered that he would entrust their care to me, and I arranged to add them on to my next clinic schedule. I had been told ahead of time that Jan was showing some changes in language, garbling her speech. The hope was that she was having some psychosomatic manifestation of stress. However, when Jan and her husband, Rick, walked into the clinic, two things became apparent: These were open and fun-loving souls, the type of people I get along with best; and she had a serious aphasia. There was no way she could be "faking" this problem. She was, at age 46, too young for stroke and unfortunately just about the right age for a brain tumor. We immediately arranged for her to have an urgent brain scan. I told them not to go home before completing this test.

An hour and a half after we had parted ways, my pager went off; it was the neuroradiologist on-call for the evening. He confirmed that Jan had a tumor in the brain, interfering with an area that manages language, and worse still, it looked like this tumor had been generated from an older tumor somewhere else in the body. Jan went from the radiology suite to a hospital bed to initiate a full workup. By the next afternoon, we had located three more tumors: two in the lungs, which were probably the original sources, and one in the liver. The prognosis was awful. I felt awful. The cancer had been there long enough to set up shop in three different places throughout Jan's body. Even if we could take the brain tumor out without disturbing Jan's speaking ability, the other tumors indicated that the cancer already had a huge head start on us.

I hadn't even gone to dinner with these people, and I was already hating the idea of losing Jan. She was one of those rare people who have a golden light emanating from them, and I felt good basking in it. To make matters worse, Rick and Jan had three children ranging in age from tween to not-even-done-with-high-school. Someone needed to explain to them why their mother was in the hospital. I was that person.

They gave me their full attention in a little waiting room down the hall from their mother's hospital bed. I told them that she was going to have surgery to remove a brain tumor, and that I was afraid things would not go well overall, because the other tumors would lead to her death in as few as six months. Tom Neuman calls that "hanging the black crepe." It's not easy to hang black crepe in a room with children, and somehow even more disconcerting to do so when those children seem to be absorbing the news quietly and with some compassion for how awkward the speaker feels. As is my nature, I tried to bring up the positive side of the situation. Knowing that they enjoyed taking scuba diving trips together, I said that their mother should be able to go back to Bonaire with them after her surgery, and it would probably be better to make that dive trip sooner than later. I suggested that their parents could probably use more help than usual around the house because they might be busy with lots of medical appointments. To my surprise, they asked some reasonable questions about their mother's condition and then thanked me for telling them. This family did not descend through levels of denial, anger, or bargaining; they concentrated instead on what could be enjoyed right now and what action could be taken right now.

The hospital staff were completely undone by this case, hating the grim reality of Jan's prognosis, but also inspired by the family. After the surgery, Rick and Jan invited the hospital staff involved to their house for dinner. Having been well schooled by Fairy Godmother Judie by that time, I knew to say, "Yes, thank you, I'll be there with bells on." That night, I was surprised that of all the doctors and nurses who'd been invited, I was the only one at the dinner table. This time around, I felt strongly that it would be easier to get to know this family and eventually mourn their loss with them than to stay at arm's length.

More than a decade has now passed since that dinner. The youngest of the children is in law school, and the oldest is expecting a second child. *Jan regularly babysits her grandson.*

After the surgical resection of the brain tumor, Rick had gotten right to work on seeking cutting-edge chemotherapeutic alternatives. Jan is the poster child for a drug from AstraZeneca. It shrank her thoracic tumors and they have not dared come back. I was clearly wrong about her prognosis, and gladly so. Their family, including extended family, adopted me and have provided me with generous friendship, hospitality that extends to the Hawai'ian Islands where they have vacation homes, and an entirely different outlook on the doctor–patient relationship. I am the only one among us with a medical degree, but I am sure they have taken more care of me than I have of them. They were there for me as I was going through my divorce, making sure that I ate, offering a restorative house to rent by the beach after I moved out of the marital domicile. They have also introduced me to other friends, like Bill, who have taught me important lessons.

Some physicians recognize that we have a strength in communication, as opposed to technical or surgical innovation. My father taught me: Admit what you don't know, listen, and offer what you do have expertise in, considering the options aloud and sharing your logic. I acknowledge frequently that in the field of dementia, there are no cures and there won't be cures in the next few years. The objective has to shift to creative problem solving for caregivers. Many days, the best we can do for caregivers is to give them a place to vent their frustration.

This enhances the trust patients and their families will extend and allows them to participate in the decision making. When we work out the care plan together, even if I'm in the leadership role, this collaboration actually takes some of the stress off my shoulders. When we all understand that the new medication may not work, and we all agree on what the target symptoms are and for how long we will try this out, I don't find myself feeling guilty if we all agree later that it did not, in fact, work.

Family education can be difficult. Aside from emotional duress, their sheer exhaustion can set up a barrier to comprehension and prescriptive action. I've experienced this phenomenon myself, when competing in swim–run biathlons in San Diego during my neurology residency training. We'd begin with a half-mile swim in the ocean, then emerge, lace up running shoes and carry on down the beach and back. A radiology professor had encouraged me to try this out, and we laughed about how I would typically pass John in the water, but then he'd steadily run me down and pass me halfway through the run section. After the first couple of times, I noted that I was having trouble during the transition, losing time in fumbling with my shoes to get each one on the correct foot, then tying the laces. When we debriefed Monday morning with the weekend's brain MRI scans dangling before us, John explained that he figured we lose at least 10 IQ points due to loss of core temperature and hypoglycemia during the swim. It's a perfect example of a situation where the intent is clear, the objective is seemingly simple, the distractions are few, and yet the brain is unable (not unwilling!) to coordinate the activity.

This particular analogy was resurrected many years later when I met the wife of a patient with Primary Progressive Aphasia, which had sniped out his language skills, then led to lapses in behavior and comportment. Katherine had, at the age of 41, qualified to compete in the Ironman championships in Kona, Hawai'i. As a journalist aiming to increase public awareness of frontotemporal dementias after her husband's diagnosis, Katherine has worked with me, and we have become great friends in the process.

I resolved to cheer her on in Kona for the Ironman event, and through a happy chance meeting in the street, I got a job as a volunteer in the main transition area for the racers. The supervisors for the area told us that the athletes would call out what they wanted as they ran by, and our job was simple: to extend cups of water, Gatorade, or ice as requested by each passing athlete. However, the physics of the situation complicates things. We are standing still, the athletes are moving, and the items in the cups will be incited to move in various directions, depending on how the athlete in motion contacts the stationary *kokua*, or volunteer support worker. By the time all the competitors had converted from swim gear to biking gear, we volunteers were thoroughly soaked and sticky with Gatorade.

It occurred to me that it felt like being in the Memory Clinic—with physicians trying to impart medical information during a crisis and just having those words wash back at us in a misunderstood jumble. At the end of the event, I asked Katherine and her Iron-galpals if there's a better way for the volunteers to hand out the cups. They laughed at the thought that they were in charge of knowing what they wanted. The athletes have a vague idea that they need something, but they need so many things, some of which are not on offer, and they're trying to transition to the next phase of the triathlon in less than a minute, so there is no truly effective way to communicate during that blur of time. I realized that this is what caregivers are trying to achieve around dementia.

Most people these days have a sophisticated grasp on how the body works, but when they are unwell or are frightened for the sake of someone else, their ability to understand the illness and the treatment is impaired. Or they have difficulty retaining the information long enough to make a decision. Some might call this denial, others an aversion to the present and imminent suffering. Neither is wrong or "bad," and both are entirely human.

In these cases, the physician or someone else from the health care team needs to be able to explain what is happening in a digestible way, filtering out the unnecessary and distracting details, devising analogies that are individualized to the listener's context, or laying a basic foundation that can be retained and then built upon whenever we revisit the subject. I may not find the cure for Alzheimer's disease before I retire, but I think I can and have helped caregivers feel better about what they are doing and how they are doing it.

12

CURRENTLY IN THE DOCTOR'S BLACK BAG

The top priority at my clinic is to help Alzheimer's families figure out the goals of treatment. There are so many things on the to-do list for a full-time caregiver that doctors can guide decision making about medications by focusing on a general shortlist of goals for each day. Once the patient has moderate to severe symptoms of a dementia, what is most important to achieve on a daily basis? The following list of simple goals usually elicits agreement with family members:

- To feel safe
- To feel pain-free
- To participate in a meaningful activity, which may not be coherent conversation with another person
- To feel loved

This happens to be an application of the Four Intentions of Buddhism to each patient's circumstances, and it's a given that those circumstances will change over time.

For some patients to feel safe, medication may be necessary to ensure they don't suffer from frightening delusions or chronic arthritic pain.

Facilitating a loved one's participation in meaningful activities may require a huge mind-shift to accept that a parent has been reduced from having a productive career to making something ornamental out of clay or beads. It can be excruciatingly painful for family caregivers to make this shift. Calculating the degree of difficulty of a task so that the patient still has as much autonomy and engagement as possible may require some creative problem solving if the patient cannot learn new activities or lacks the motor coordination to participate in former hobbies. On a day-to-day basis, the patient may have some very confused days alternating with relatively lucid ones. Regardless of whether it is a good day or a tougher one, the goal is to help him succeed at having some pleasurable moments. Sitting in the quiet company of a beloved household pet can be significant and just as important as participating in a hobby. The caregiver's challenge is to remain flexible enough to share in even the smallest of successes.

Those patients who wander away from home base may be in search of some meaningful stimulation, and this may create a dilemma for caregivers. It is important for caregivers to feel they are promoting as much autonomy as possible, but where are the boundaries? An anonymous American judge's definition of freedom may be most applicable: "Your right to swing your arms ends just where the other man's nose begins." The patient's activity must not bring harm to himself or others. Individual communities may have varying levels of resources to sustain someone who is having behavioral problems. If the patient's behaviors are frightening to others, he may be safest if his range is limited to those who know him well and are willing to help. For the patient to be safe, those around him need to feel safe too. Global positioning systems (GPS) are becoming more widely used to track dementia patients who wander. Families may differ over the ethical dilemma of tracking patients without their consent. But GPS can prevent panic when trying to locate patients who can walk and run or catch a cab on their own.

The last item on the list—to feel loved—can be the hardest or the easiest to accomplish, depending upon the history between the caregiver and the patient, and the patient's symptoms. Some patients become much more affectionate with dementia and treasure a hug or being held. In these cases, caregivers may need to accept the fact that the patient will obtain this kind of affection from other people. Conversely, some patients become less comfortable with close contact, and caregivers who favor a "touchy-feely" approach may have to switch to a more verbal way of expressing their positive feelings. A sense of peaceful acceptance and companionship may be transmitted most clearly through just having some quiet downtime near the patient. I will frequently prescribe time for the caregiver to let go of the nagging, quizzing, coaching role, in order to achieve a sense of calm stillness with a loved one. I can't imagine how awful it would be to see dismay over my every failure on the face of a companion. Although the patient may not be able to verbalize what he or she is feeling or needing, in most cases, the ability to pick up on the stress someone has brought into the room remains intact, and the patient often reacts negatively to it.

Caregivers find peace of mind if they know that everything that can be done for the patient is being done. What can we do while the course of dementia slowly unfolds? First, I'd ensure that the diagnostic evaluation is complete and up to current standards. Currently, there is no blood test that can confirm the diagnosis of a dementia. When a doctor orders blood work as part of the diagnostic evaluation, the purpose is to check for reversible causes of cognitive impairment. We routinely check for syphilis and vitamin B12 deficiency, because both are reversible conditions that can sometimes masquerade as neuro-degenerative dementia.

When the onset of symptoms is rapid and related to a viral illness, a spinal tap or lumbar puncture is added to the diagnostic work-up for dementia. That way, the cerebrospinal fluid can be examined to rule out various infections, such as a meningitis caused by a virus or fungus. Just as importantly, there is increasing evidence that the spinal fluid can reflect the abnormal protein profile harbored by the brain. While patients in North America are leery about letting someone poke a long needle into their backs, it is common practice in Sweden, where patients have been taught by clinicians and researchers that a lumbar puncture is part of a thorough work-up for dementia. It may even turn out to be a way to predict the risk level for memory loss at a point before it is irreversible. Impressively, international collaborations have formed to share the cerebrospinal fluid obtained from lumbar puncture procedures. The labs follow clear, harmonized guidelines so that they are drawing the same amount of fluid from each patient at a consistent time of day and can share the samples with each other to increase sample size when they run experiments. Cerebrospinal fluid testing is expensive, costing up to a thousand dollars per patient.

From the way television shows portray doctors and science, the general public has learned to expect several layers of laboratory and imaging evidence before the doctor arrives at a definitive conclusion. The lay public then, understandably but fruitlessly, inquires about testing for prevention and for diagnosis. In memory clinics, clinicians believe that with a full history, some evidence on cognitive testing, and neuroimaging, we can tell a patient what type of dementia we need to manage.

The million-dollar question is, "What are we looking for on those brain pictures?" In the 1990s, the advent and wide distribution of computerized tomography (CT) scanning and magnetic resonance imaging (MRI) scanning greatly advanced neurology. Most emergency rooms have a CT scanner, which quickly reveals bleeding in the brain, skull fractures, or brain tumors. MRI scans generally take longer to obtain but can deliver a great deal of high-resolution information about the structures inside the brain. Unfortunately, both CT and MRI scanning are more telling when the person has lived into the middle of his illness; these images can be far less helpful if we are trying to make an early diagnosis.

Currently neuroimaging is used to detect brain tumors or bleeding or loss of brain tissue in the brain, but another important role for neuroimaging may be to identify the presence of abnormal proteins that cause dementia. Researchers are racing to discover ways of tracking the abnormal accumulation of proteins in living, breathing patients before they progress too far into illness. For instance, we can radioactively label amyloid—the abnormal protein associated with Alzheimer's disease—then look for that signal using a PET (positron emission tomography) scanner. A measure that corresponds with the illness in a specific and time-sensitive manner is referred to as a biomarker. Radioactive labels that stick to abnormal protein deposits in the brain and abnormal protein that has leaked from the brain into cerebrospinal fluid are biomarkers under development that may be helpful to our clinical needs. Doctors intend to use this type of testing to diagnose which type of protein the treatment should target. One way of treating a dementia is to stop the aggregation of the abnormal proteins. Many researchers have been investigating anti-amyloid interventions, and biomarkers that measure amyloid are used to detect the efficacy of any candidate intervention. Being able to use radiotracers or other biomarkers to locate and quantify the abnormal proteins associated with dementia has terrific implications as a diagnostic tool and as a way to track whether an intervention under study is proving useful against a particular protein.

The next few years will tell if the radiotracers designed to signal amyloid proteinopathy can go into routine use for diagnosis of Alzheimer's disease. The use of these radiotracers in PET scanners has been considered too expensive and technically demanding for prime-time clinical use, but it will soon become available more widely, at least in the United States. Because of its cost, countries practicing socialized medicine are more likely to utilize this imaging method for research purposes than as a tool for routine clinical use. This type of imaging would then function as a test for whether a target region has been engaged by a candidate treatment, but it is not likely to create new treatment strategies on its own.

Studies using amyloid tracers have raised burning questions. If a patient doesn't have any memory complaints now, but his amyloid PET scan shows a moderate amount of positive signal, how long will it be before he shows signs of Alzheimer's disease? Will he even get Alzheimer's disease? Is a PET scan showing a high level of amyloid a predictor for Alzheimer's disease, or is this negotiable? So far, only 5% of participants without cognitive impairment but high amyloid scan levels have gone on to develop cognitive impairment within the following year. Does this mean we've found an early-alert mechanism? Or does it mean that the amyloid detected by the radiotracer is not the cause of a person's outwardly trackable decline? Keep an eye peeled for the answers! My own work has extended to checking out whether amyloid plays a role in dementias other than Alzheimer's disease when patients have lived past 70.

The search for other, easier-to-assess biomarkers continues. One candidate is the lens or the retina. If this could be examined visually, without having to take a sample to view under the microscope, it would be even more convenient for patients.

The mainstay of current dementia care with pharmaceuticals addresses behavior and mood, as opposed to stopping the illness. These medications are "borrowed" from the arsenal used to treat primary psychiatric illnesses. For instance, if the patient seems sad or tearful and is ruminating on negative thoughts after a diagnosis of dementia, we will try antidepressants. The rules of prescribing generally do not differ among types of dementia, be it Alzheimer's or dementia with Lewy bodies or frontotemporal or vascular dementia. The one exception is that patients suffering from dementia with Lewy bodies and Parkinson's disease may be very vulnerable to the adverse effects of antipsychotic medications.

There are times when patients who are given to angry, aggressive episodes due to their dementia require a combination of medication and behavioral techniques. Of course we can "snow" a patient—that is, knock him or her out with a sedative—but this raises controversy. It may enable the caregiver to get a restful sleep overnight, but the trade-off for the patient is fewer hours of the day spent as awake and alert as possible. The behavioral strategy taught to me by Dr. Dmytro Rewilak, a colleague in psychology at Baycrest, begins with asking questions like "What leads to the behavior?," "What exactly is the behavior?," and "What are the consequences of the behavior?" Interestingly, the answers often reveal variables that the caregiver *can* control to reduce the unwanted behavior.

For example, if opening the oven door creates agitation and conflict, maybe it's worth not opening the oven door when the patient is in the kitchen or within earshot. Using the microwave or the toaster oven instead may markedly diminish the frequency of the upset. In cases where the trigger is unavoidable, caregivers may need to come up with a way to distract the patient from noticing the trigger stimulus.

Making careful, objective observations can lead to an important shift in perception. For example, caregivers often report that the patient is "anxious." If I can remember to practice what I preach, I ask what statements or actions from the patient indicate that anxiety instead of automatically writing a prescription for an anxiolytic medication. In the case of frontotemporal dementia, patients may look obsessive-compulsive, repeating an action that was once purposeful until it is now purposeless, like opening and closing drawers. If the patient's sign of anxiety is opening and closing drawers, I then ask if it's accompanied by crying or upset. Is the patient looking for something? Often the patient is not showing any emotion. In those cases, the caregiver and I may agree that the patient may be engaged in repetitive actions, but he or she isn't actually anxious. The patient may be seeking some sort of stimulating activity. Instead of prescribing a sedative to calm anxiety, I can suggest that the drawer be modified so that it opens and closes quietly.

Examining the consequences of the unwanted behavior can help identify ways in which that behavior is being positively reinforced. Most of us believe that yelling or otherwise showing our displeasure can keep the patient from doing something. But, in fact, that expression of displeasure may be interpreted by the patient as a way to interact with you, without a value of good or bad assigned. Buddhist teacher Thich Nhat Hanh has observed that a problem is more solvable when we (in this case, the caregivers) stop judging what is wrong or right, in favor of trying to be more skillful in the art of living together. Applying this concept to problem solving as a caregiver may reduce some of the insult perceived in patients' unwanted behaviors.

Generally, any reaction to a behavior reinforces it, if the actor's goal is to be provocative. Patients don't mean to make others angry; I believe they're just trying to connect to the people around them. Behavioral therapists have reframed "behavioral disturbance" as "responsive behaviors," which leads to an investigation of what is causing a patient to behave a certain way. The assumption is that the patient is communicating a need that can't be verbalized. Many patients with dementia retain the ability to understand the emotional tenor of the room, even if they can't respond verbally, and being around a caregiver who is upset disturbs them. Wherever possible, do not let unwanted behaviors escalate upset. When the cause is unclear, it's better to calmly distract the patient into doing something else more productive, meaningful, or at least sustainable. This is often very, very difficult to do, and takes large measures of mindfulness and equanimity.

The next step is to determine if medication is intended more to benefit the patient or the caregiver. Sometimes, we need to sedate the patient in order for the caregiver to get some rest. Ideally, we could determine what's causing any difficult behaviors and then address the cause, but there are times when the problem has persisted too long, and we need to buy some time to do a better job of investigating causes and honing the intervention. Through discussing the motivations for each new medication, caregivers can make the best-informed decisions on behalf of the patient. Sometimes the caregiver will prefer to work with the behavior rather than administer more medication, if it is understood that the behavior is not a sign of distress from the patient.

Patients who refuse to bathe create a major challenge for their caregivers. Medications that have sedative properties may succeed in making the patient more drowsy, but that does not always translate to more cooperative behavior. In fact, the treating physician must evaluate at times whether making the patient half-asleep *increases* agitation. Caregivers may have to settle for infrequent bathing of the patient. Or they can be creative about ways to get grooming done, for instance regular trips to the patient's favorite beautician, sitting in the hot tub, or going for a dip in the lake, as opposed to submitting to a formal shower. Another option is to save the caregiver from having to be the Bad Guy Bather. We can get a personal support worker to handle the bathing, if the patient can tolerate having a stranger attend to him or her. I usually stress that the caregiver has enough to do without having to play the role of the Bad Guy in the patient's life. That's a job better delegated to a trained professional.

Dementia and Alzheimer's patients may confuse day and night, and this can wreak havoc on the entire household. Included in this category of behavioral disturbance is "sundowning." In my clinic, we refer to the onset of confusion with the transition from daylight to sunset as "sundowning," but in the literature, any daytime disorientation may also be called sundowning. If the confusion is truly limited to that transition time, the family can consider several options. They can improve the lighting conditions using automatic timers to brighten up the home. They can also assess the impact of other events at that time of day that may not be related to daylight: Is there a sudden return home by several household members, which could be jarring to the patient? A change-over of hired companions that doesn't go smoothly? A sudden increase in the noise level in the environment that can cause confusion? Acetylcholinesterase inhibitors can sometimes help with this difficulty. They are generally administered in the morning with breakfast, and may help patients' alertness through the daylight hours.

Patients who reverse day and night can disrupt the sleep of their caregivers. The main goal of medical interventions, whether pharmacologic or behavioral, is to routinize daytime wakefulness for patients and to set them up to be tired and ready to sleep at night, on the same schedule as the rest of the household. This can require a different type of routine if the primary caregiver works the graveyard shift. We coach the family to keep the patient awake and actively engaged in some appropriate activity, perhaps supervised at a day program, NOT napping during the day if sleep is inconsistent or short-lived during the night.

Sedative medications (which include some antidepressants, some antipsychotics, and some medications specifically indicated for insomnia) help to establish what time of day should be bedtime. These medications for sleep do not work consistently over the long term, however, so it's important to make sure the environmental signals are reinforcing bedtime once the brain is getting used to a regular routine. The keys to success are to ensure that consistent signals denote the time of day, and to make the environment conducive to peaceful rest. We have found that some patients who seem not to respond to nighttime sleeping medications have been receiving medications to sleep during the day.

Treatment can be complicated as physicians take aim at the cognitive changes due to dementia. Adverse effects from a drug may worsen cognitive ability while calming a difficult behavior. Sometimes I have to pose a tough question to the caregiver: Does that caregiver prefer peaceful afternoons at home, or a more awake patient still attempting the newspaper crossword puzzle but unsuccessfully, due to restless agitation? Dementia with Lewy bodies and Alzheimer's disease both feature a shortage of acetylcholine, but in DLB that deficit more markedly affects the area of the brain that keeps a person awake and alert (brain stem). This challenge to the brain stem can allow a patient to look like he is having a few lucid days at a time, followed precipitously by very confused days. Of course this is very unsettling for family members who may welcome the lucidity as a lifting of the illness—until the confusion returns. The family's expectations can roller coaster until they get a good medical explanation for how DLB works.

The cholinesterase-inhibitor medications available for Alzheimer's disease can help smooth out those fluctuations in alertness. If a fairly early stage of DLB has been diagnosed, the patient can often show great benefit with the cholinesterase inhibitor. Unfortunately for both Alzheimer's disease and DLB patients, this type of medication does not actually add acetylcholine to the brain. Medications that do this are rife with adverse effects because the body has many uses for acetylcholine, and to have all of those functions keyed up leads to heavy mucus production, profuse sweating, and other intolerable discomforts.

In both Alzheimer's and DLB, the patient is losing the ability to produce his own acetylcholine, a chemical that the brain uses as the currency to transfer information. Brain chemicals that act as the currency for neuron-to-neuron transactions are a link between changes in the brain's proteostasis and the outward manifestation of dementia. This doesn't happen in the mild cognitive impairment stage of Alzheimer's disease—it seems to occur a year or more later, at around the time the person loses independent function. During mild cognitive impairment, some have detected a signal that the brain is in a compensatory mode, kicking up production of acetylcholine to make up for the impending deficiency.

Cholinesterase inhibitors allow patients to get more mileage out of the acetylcholine they can still make on their own. But at a certain point in the illness, the brain is not making enough acetylcholine, and it does not matter how much cholinesterase inhibitor is tossed at the system, since there is no substrate with which the drug can work. Cholinesterase inhibitors, therefore, are a good example of a symptomatic drug, as opposed to a disease-modifying drug.

The world would be an easier place if acetylcholine pills could make up for the progressive deficit in the brain, but acetylcholine's activity in the body below the neck runs counter to its role in the brain. Whereas the brain is generally activated and memory relies upon good acetylcholine flow between the hippocampus and other cross-referencing file bins within the brain, a blast of acetylcholine to the body can cause the over-secetion crisis described on the previous page. The symptoms of an acetylcholine overdose will be familiar to anyone who has overdosed on medication for myasthenia gravis or encountered nerve gas or farming organophosphates: weakness that makes it hard to breathe, and oversecretion of bodily fluids like saliva and sweat. There's a mnemonic for the opposite situation, a disabling blockade of acetylcholine receptors, that always makes me think of *Alice in Wonderland*: "blind as a bat (pupils can't focus), dry as a bone, red as a beet (Queen of Hearts?), *mad as a hatter*." Certainly we're all more comfortable living within the middle range of acetylcholine levels. The phrase "cholinergic deficit" is particular to Alzheimer's disease and one line of therapy for it. In Alzheimer's disease, brain cells are not making acetylcholine anymore, but there is enough acetylcholine in the rest of the body.

The challenge of treating Alzheimer's patients specifically for their brains' cholinergic deficit is to find an agent that can get into the brain and act inside it, without initiating the debilitating systemic effects described above. Agents that directly activate acetylcholine receptors have been too toxic for patients in the past. The huge breakthrough of the early 1990s was the advent of the cholinesterase inhibitor. The idea was elegant: Don't add more acetylcholine through an oral medication that will cause cholinergic crisis systemically; instead, slow down the enzymes that break acetylcholine down in the brain. In this way, the cholinesterase inhibitors get more mileage out of the acetylcholine made by the brain. This strategy is great for making the treatment tolerable to patients, but it's not terribly effective once the brain's production of acetylcholine has declined too much to give a good minimum flow of acetylcholine.

The mechanism of action of acetylcholinesterase inhibitors was a new concept for drug approval. The fight to get Health Canada or the Food and Drug Administration to approve a drug that was not yet a cure but could help patients in the early stages of Alzheimer's disease required a new way of thinking about what drugs are for and what's worth insurance coverage. Antibiotics are not to slow the progression of disease; they are to cure the infection. The concept of a symptomatic treatment, as opposed to something that will modify or cure the disease, was hard for everyone to buy into at first.

My first doctor-patient with Alzheimer's disease was a retired family practitioner who understood that he had progressive memory impairment. I was very impressed to learn over our visits that after his wife had passed on, Bob was reunited with a family friend. The doctor-widower began a new, long-distance relationship with this woman. Bob's dementia was not a deal-breaker for this new partner. He, understandably, wanted to impress her. There is no woman who wakes up in the morning saying, "I do NOT want to be swept off my feet today." So my doctor-patient took his medication, a cholinesterase inhibitor approved by the FDA for treatment of Alzheimer's disease. And after the first level of dosing, he felt sharper of mind, so he took the next level of dosing. Most physicians hold their prescriptions at that second dose, but Bob believed more would be better. This was a mistake. It caused him to faint. This was also the time when sildenafil (also known as Viagra®) first became available. The same logic was used by the doctor-patient for all his medications, ultimately inducing a cardiac arrhythmia. They say doctors make the worst patients. I won't comment on that, but I do know it's only human to call upon your own experience in problem solving, and that dementia can get in the way of making those connections wisely.

Some interventions that stave off the onset of dementia can help optimize a patient's function despite his dementia diagnosis: These are exercise, diet, and sleep. The treatment role of physical activity is still unclear; evidence supports the theory that regular physical activity works more as a preventive measure than as a treatment for dementia. Most researchers agree that physical activity stimulates neuronal remodeling, bolsters cognitive reserve, and staves off obesity and other metabolic syndromes that render an individual more vulnerable to dementia. But the same mechanisms of action that achieve the preventive benefits also "tune up" brain performance in general. Enhanced blood and oxygen flow to a dementia-injured brain, attention to the appropriate glucose levels, and reduction of hindrances to cerebral blood flow can't but help us compensate for cognitive impairment.

Sleep is very important for both patient and caregiver. We are learning more all the time about what the brain does while we sleep or rest, not just perchance to dream. Only mammals and songbirds have complex sleep architecture, descending through several stages repeatedly throughout one night's sleep, and that complexity of sleep places us at an advantage to learn!

Time to consolidate during sleep what you've experienced daily can serve as cross-referencing for the filing of information you'd like to access at a later date. You don't do this during all sleep hours—it is specific to one stage of sleep! Consider each new experience or episode of your day's activities to be a separate Post-it note. Envision them stuck all over one wall, a desktop, your computer monitor, and overrunning your sock drawer. Consolidation is like sorting that multitude of square pieces of paper into categories and cross-referenced stacks. Another function of sleep is to allow us full alertness during the day so that we can do a more complete job of committing experiences to those Post-it notes. If the note is written in the equivalent of gibberish, no filing system will be able to accommodate it.

Another intervention that is seldom regarded as treatment is placement in a long-term-care facility. If family members are unable to provide a safe, happy, healthy, and loving environment at home, a long-term care facility with well-trained staff in good numbers may be therapeutic. Patients with advanced dementia can thrive in a well-structured environment that assigns appropriate expectations and promotes positive interactions throughout the day. When families are no longer able to provide care to the patient by themselves, the patient may have to move into a facility. Sometimes this occurs despite every good intention on the part of the caregiver, but a caregiver's illness or injury may render him unable to provide the same level of care to the patient as before.

I encourage families to look for innovative, client-centered homes. They do exist. Colleagues had invited me to visit day programs in Hong Kong while I was there for a conference. The one that stands out most in my memory was across the road from a horseracing track. To satisfy its public service commitment, the Royal Hong Kong Jockey Club had committed a percentage of the gambling proceeds to fund a state-of-the-art day seniors' center for patients with Alzheimer's disease. It was like the Ritz-Carlton Hotel of day programs.

The important thing was not the newness of the furniture. The directors had consulted with gerontologists, geriatric psychiatrists, and neurologists to design an environment that would set each client up for success. The common areas were appointed as if they were dining rooms and sitting rooms of the era when the clients would have been in their thirties. The recreational room looked like a place a client would have expected to sit down to an afternoon of mahjong with friends. For residents in the attached long-term-care facility, the drawers had see-through plastic fronts, so there was no guessing game as to where an article of clothing might be kept. Labels and signage were discreet yet perfectly placed to help direct clients to where they wanted to go.

An outdoor terrace housed a garden supervised by a recreational therapist. The layout accommodated those who needed a safe place to walk around or pace without running into barriers or other clients, but also without feeling locked in like a prisoner.

There was also a Quiet Room, where therapists worked to

discover what non-pharmacological interventions might suit a patient who was feeling confused and agitated. Inside that room were soft lighting, a massage chair, and items of multiple textures, especially for clients who would do best with simple stimulation and could no longer enjoy a conversation or a hobby. This was a model for the rest of us! They've more recently moved on to a cyber seniors' center—as the Boomers age, they will be more comfortable with electronics and robot technology, and it looks like Hong Kong is ready.

I was attracted to the job at Baycrest in Toronto, despite having to give up my fair Southern California weather, because it is another well-supported, innovative care facility for seniors. Patients with frontotemporal dementia are frequently too physically healthy and behaviorally disturbed or incontinent to be eligible for a standard day program for patients with late-onset dementia. The staff identified the preference of frontotemporal dementia caregivers for day program respite instead of caregiver support groups. In many cases, the caregiver is so busy at providing care that there's no time to find someone else to watch the patient so that the primary caregiver can leave home to attend a meeting. Within a very short period of time, the Memory Clinic staff worked with the existing seniors' day center staff (we already had two programs going, one for cognitively impaired older patients and another for physically frail ones) to formulate a first-time proposal to start a frontotemporal dementia day program at Baycrest. Because of the institution's strong reputation in working out and then disseminating best practices in elder care, the Ministry of Health granted Joyce Lagunoff, then director of the seniors' center, the money without batting an eyelash. Joyce continues to pass it off as no big effort on her part, but we have regularly gotten calls from other Canadian provinces, the U.S., and Europe to learn how we set this up. I'd say it was the serendipity of good timing and being at the right place with like-minded people.

Despite this success, Baycrest and other multi-purpose facilities for elder care that include long-term care and hospice can be feared by patients as their final destination. I recall in my first few months on the job at Baycrest, a bit giddy with all the resources available for my clinic patients and for my research interests, that one clinic patient had a very different view of what was going on within our four walls. She was extremely anxious about our appointment and seemed ready to bolt out the door. Trying to put her at ease, I pushed my papers aside, put down my pen, and asked what we could do to make her feel more comfortable. She revealed, "They've brought me to Baycrest!"

"Yes," I replied with a smile, "and it's a great place to get help."

"No! My family brought me here to die!"

My heart sank. What a horrible feeling that must be. And I think it wasn't so much the fact that she was going to die that was as terrifying as the thought of being abandoned to face the end alone. Luckily, I could reassure her that our schedule for the day entailed a two-hour visit and then I would send her home with her children in time to beat their parking meter. What is a nursing home, though? To many people, it is a place you go to die. We need to work on that image.

It is because of the stigma of the long-term-care facility (previously known as a nursing home) that many families are instead trying to place their loved ones with dementia into retirement homes. The intention is to surround the patient with healthy peers, and there is often a deal made with the retirement home officials that privately arranged caregiver personnel will be sent to the facility to provide hands-on care for the patient daily so as not to tax whatever minimal supervision is already in place for the other, more independently living retirees. This is an expensive option and it can work. But it can also lead to conflict within the family about what is the better path. One could argue that the professionals at a long-term care facility have had more training on how to work with a cognitively impaired patient than the personal support workers available to service retirement homes. The Alzheimer's Association/Alzheimer Society have made it their duty to offer continuing education to personal support workers to bridge the gap in knowledge between them and registered nurses, but some patients are especially challenging as their course of illness progresses, and it is probably most helpful to ask the treating physician and case manager for advice on what type of facility would be best for each individual case.

My next effort in education will be to bring together a creative team to design educational materials for children who live in a household where there is a person with dementia. There is an entirely different set of stressors for children than for their parents, and I think the time has come to empower them to participate in ensuring that the patient feels safe, happy, and pain-free. In fact, I suspect that children can be more flexible in what types of interactions they can have with patients to provide good company—they are closer to the concept of "play" than are adults.

The impact of dementia differs from household to household. Although two patients may have the same density of memory loss, in one house, it could be a godsend that the patient no longer has the memory that fueled a post-traumatic stress disorder. In another house, the memory loss might keep the patient from continuing his role as caregiver to his spouse, who is incapacitated by severe arthritis. In the first case, medications to improve memory function are not warranted. In the second case, the family is more motivated to fight the cognitive decline. Since we have no silver bullet for curing dementing illness, the management of these patients arises from a dialogue between doctors and families about what is essentially damage control.

My colleagues and I are not helpless against dementia—we have the means to address its symptoms, albeit mainly through the use of off-label drugs (which are explained in the next chapter). More importantly, we have the means to reduce stress for the caregivers.

13

NEW AVENUES OF RESEARCH

When I meet new people, their first question after learning what I do for a living is typically, "So have they found something to treat that yet?" Many labs are working from myriad angles to solve dementia. Upwards of US$2 billion have been invested in Alzheimer's disease treatment trials that unfortunately did not bear fruit. As a result, there is no cure available on the shelf for even the most common dementia, Alzheimer's disease, yet much of the last decade's research has helped us to understand how the brain is getting into trouble. And that will lead to treatment.

One challenge to treating dementia effectively is to develop interventions that work at each of the stages of the illness. What works at the beginning may be too little too late toward the end of the course of illness. And the circle of people who can be described as "patients" is wide. It can include people who are worried that a strong family history of illness puts them at high risk to develop dementia; those who have been newly diagnosed with mild symptoms; those whose diagnosis may have been delayed so that they now have even more brain pathology to struggle with; and those who have lost so much independent function that they need something that will reverse the illness and its cumulative consequences, not just something that will stabilize their current condition.

At this point doctors are convinced that treating patients earlier will garner a positive response, whereas acting late may not work, at least in that we cannot restore cognitive ability "after the horse is out of the barn." Admittedly, this has led to some confusion for researchers in terms of whether they should be focusing on developing preventive measures as opposed to formulating treatment for those already diagnosed. The majority of candidate drugs have not worked for those at moderate or later stages of illness, but there is hope that they could work for patients with very early, low levels of abnormal protein build-up.

Because different proteins cause different types of dementia, some early interventions will be designed to take aim at specific protein abnormalities. Frontotemporal dementia patients do not have amyloid plaques, so their therapy to stop progression of their illness will differ from that of Alzheimer's disease patients. For a while, we weren't sure which protein abnormality caused the majority of cases of frontotemporal dementia, but now we have a suspect, TDP-43, and thus we can be more specific about developing therapies for that illness.

At the opposite end of the course of dementia, if there's a final common step to the abnormal proteins' irreversible damage to the brain, a drug or procedure that stops that final process ought to work for Alzheimer's disease, for frontotemporal dementia, for DLB, and for Parkinson's disease. Although this gives researchers a second window of opportunity for intervention, the most effective timing of treatment to preserve a person's quality of life would be earlier in the disease process, before the final common pathway. Midway through the illness, clearing half of the proteinopathy might stop further progression, but once on the final common stage, the objective would have to include both halting the disease process and restoring brain disconnections. That latter part of the mission might seem impossible, but researchers are calling upon the principles of plasticity discussed earlier.

Any promising modes of *prevention* have been discovered as a by-product of their failure to treat dementia. Resveratrol is an example of this storyline. Resveratrol, naturally present in grapes and pomegranates, can inhibit beta-amyloid deposition but doesn't do much for a patient after a critically damaging mass of beta-amyloid has already been laid down. Most laypeople understand that antioxidants can be weapons against aging, but not many understand that once a patient with dementia has become moderately disabled, taking antioxidant supplements like vitamin E or eating more antioxidant foods (blueberries, for example) will not reverse the illness.

Neuropathologist Ian Mackenzie, at the University of British Columbia, noted a particular pattern of abnormal protein deposits as he sifted through brain tissue donated by patients with frontotemporal dementia. Working closely with neurologists from his team, he's generated descriptive papers that link courses of illness (types of symptoms and speed of mortality) to the abnormal protein variations accumulated in the patients' brains. The next step in his work has been to work closely with geneticists, like Rosa Rademakers at the Mayo Clinic in Rochester, to link genetic material from those autopsy samples with the protein accumulations. Rademakers, in turn, has been working with biochemists who can examine cerebrospinal fluid to look for abnormal protein production while the patient is still alive. Using evidence gleaned from the end of a patient's life has, in this way, led to ways to detect onset of the illness much earlier. Those who carry a genetic mutation related to dementia but who seem otherwise untouched by the illness are the individuals we can follow more closely to detect when and why the brain starts producing abnormal proteins.

How does one go about identifying the abnormal proteins and learning how and why they appear in the brain? We start at the end of life and work our way backward. Autopsies on the brain tell us what abnormal proteins have accumulated over the course of illness. The downside to using this evidence is that it reduces decades of disease process to the last moments. It's as if we are trying to figure out what happened at a party by examining the trash bin the next morning. Numerous empty, greasy pizza boxes, tangles of decorative crepe paper, countless empty beer and wine bottles, the stench of cigarette butts, and maybe a broken piece of furniture signify that a social event has occurred and may have gotten out of hand. But there is little to identify which invited guests actually attended, whether they arrived gradually or all on the same bus, how long they stayed, and who were the most obnoxious guests. What were they celebrating? Who failed to eject the hooligans before damage was done?

The study of detecting how abnormal proteins form and collect is called proteomics, which looks suspiciously like "the economics of proteins" made into a fancier word. Investigating dementia in this way allows for wider thinking in terms of dividing proteins into those that directly cause disease and those that increase *risk* for developing the disease. Alternatively, abnormal protein collections may arise as a by-product of some other important damaging process (as if they were innocent bystanders), as opposed to causing damage themselves.

The latest lead on how the amyloid of Alzheimer's disease enters its abnormal manufacturing phase is that prions can prompt the abnormal formation of proteins that aggregate into the clumps neuropathologists see in the brain at the end of illness. Following the analogy of the mystery party, the prion may turn out to be the host for the party. A prion is a relatively new concept, an idea that combines the principles of infectious disease, genetics, and proteomics. A prion has a smaller structure than a virus, yet it can be every bit as or more effective in causing damage, because it disables the inner workings of targeted cells. In the case of dementia, prions may initiate the premature demise of a person's brain. Nobel laureate Stan Prusiner at the University of California, San Francisco, figured out the key to how diseases like scrapie, which affects sheep, or "mad cow disease," which gained notoriety in the 1990s, spread. Those have been explained as diseases caused by prions, and neuro-degenerative diseases such as Alzheimer's disease, Parkinson's disease, and amyotrophic lateral sclerosis are shaping up to be the next identified prion diseases.

If prions are the hosts bringing abnormal proteins into an unauthorized gathering in the brain, one would expect the immune system to act as one type of bouncer to keep the riffraff from becoming brain-wreckers. This strategy may sound straightforward, but immune responses to the unwanted proteins apparently cause more damage, as opposed to kicking out the garbage in an orderly fashion. Hence, a counterintuitive theory—that the inflammatory response should be stopped in order to stave off Alzheimer's disease—was put to the test.

Non-steroidal anti-inflammatory drugs (NSAIDs) include many preparations available over the counter, such as aspirin, ibuprofen, and acetaminophen. Antioxidants, found in vitamin E and blueberries, are another form of anti-inflammatory agent. Studies with these agents have not validated the anti-inflammatory hypothesis. The tempting piece of information that ignited that line of investigation was from the Baltimore Longitudinal Study of Aging: Subjects who had taken NSAIDs more than just every once in a while were less likely to develop Alzheimer's disease. Diehard supporters of this theory have argued that the wrong kinds of NSAIDs were administered in prevention trials that failed. The latest NSAID trial hypothesizes that low doses—as opposed to high doses—of anti-inflammatory medications will be beneficial for preventing Alzheimer's disease. Just as with estrogens for women, there could be a small window of opportunity during which taking NSAIDs would play a key role in preventing brain disease but not in treating dementia.

If prions are the hosts of the "dementia party," inviting abnormal proteins to gather, and the immune system is the gate-crasher at the party who compounds the damage done to the brain, there are other potential "bouncers." One of the reasons that dementia begins later in life and not in early childhood is that the brain's ability to deactivate and clear its flawed protein products falters and may be lost entirely in late life. A protein's efficacy is determined in large part by how its three-dimensional configuration fits with the rest of the cell. The abnormality in the proteins related to dementia is in the way they are folded, and this failure to follow the origami instructions needs to be "tagged and bagged" before it can cause damage to the cell. Where possible, one type of the brain's bouncers identifies the misfolded proteins and labels them accordingly for other bouncer staff to clear away. One of the impacts of aging on our cells is that the tag-and-bag bouncers lose efficiency. When that results in an unbalanced ratio between functional, desirable proteins and abnormal ones, clumping of the abnormal protein triggers the downward spiral of neurodegeneration.

As described in Chapter 8, there are diet-related ways to restore the tag-and-bag bouncers: namely, controlling insulin and calorie intake. More and more of us are updating our knowledge about the delicate balance of glucose in the body. Too much glucose too often, related to diabetes and obesity, is toxic to the brain. Additionally, one indirect effect of hyperglycemia on dementia is to reduce the clearance of rogue amyloid. The balance is tricky, however, since the opposite condition, hypoglycemia, can also be detrimental to the brain! Accordingly, manufacturers of medications for diabetes are racing to prove that their drug has some protective effect against Alzheimer's disease. They are searching for the exact therapeutic range of glucose control in order to rate an indication for dementia from the drug regulatory agencies.

Caloric restriction, which results in resveratrol increases, keys up cellular stress resistance, likely through several means. In the old Western movies, settlers under attack would quickly position their covered wagons into a defensive circle; caloric restriction triggers changes within the cell that effectively circle the wagons. It remains unclear how long the cell can keep its wagons circled, so there is a possibility that one might benefit from exercising calorie restriction on a recurrent and not continuous basis.

We can also reduce the percentage of failed origami products by influencing microRNAs. Researchers have discovered that microRNAs play a special role in the manufacture of proteins by a cell. DNA provides the recipe, RNA and ribosomes are a bit like sous-chefs using amino acids as their ingredients, and proteins are the dishes served. MicroRNAs fit into that kitchen as the chefs who control when and how much of a particular product is coming off the line. If the microRNAs related to a dementia's proteinopathy could be called into action, it could halt disease. Right now the microRNA intervention that looks most promising is one that increases progranulin production, which would be helpful for some patients with frontotemporal dementia.

An international approach to proteomics, led by Rick Morimoto at Northwestern University, has looked at yet another type of "bouncer" to deter undesirable proteinopathy clumps. These scientists have described "chaperone proteins" that facilitate tagging and bagging. Some researchers are working on how to stabilize or enhance the chaperones' function—like organizing shifts of parents to monitor the kids' wild house party. Dr. Gillian Bates's lab at King's College London is finding a way to amp up the chaperoning in Huntington's disease to counteract the unwanted product of that disease mutation, called Huntingtin.

Those chaperones are assigned within the mitochondrion, the cellular energy plant that was transcribed from your mother's DNA. Other medications being tried in animal models and getting to the first phase of human clinical trials are aimed at various chemical processes within the mitochondrion. Those interventions theoretically would decrease the production of toxic wastes that can build up in the cell and kill it, or at least make the mitochondrion function more efficiently. Coenzyme Q10 is an agent felt to aid impaired mitochondrial function, and it has already been recommended for amyotrophic lateral sclerosis and Parkinson's disease.

We haven't succeeded yet with drug therapies aimed against already-formed protein collections that have taken hold in the brain. Slowing down or stopping the enzymes that are activated by prions or genetic factors to make rogue proteins could also stop the decline of dementia. Alzheimer's researchers have taken particular pains to find a blocker for an enzyme called glycogen synthase kinase-3 alpha (GSK-3a), because it enables production of the rogue versions of amyloid and tau. That enzyme may also be responsible for frontotemporal dementia, because some cases are characterized by abnormal tau. Amazingly, GSK-3a is further implicated in the abnormal protein of Parkinson's disease and dementia with Lewy bodies. That protein is alpha-synuclein, which clumps into damaging Lewy bodies. By controlling this one enzyme, could we prevent several types of dementia? The optimists among us are dazzled by the potential!

How does GSK-3a do its dirty work? GSK-3a is very important to normal protein manufacture and processing in the neuron, and there's an optimal range of activity. The relationship between GSK-3a and Alzheimer's proteinopathy is complex. GSK-3a may be activated at normal levels until beta-amyloid has formed. Under the influence of a small amount of beta-amyloid, GSK-3a activity perks up, which then increases the erroneous manufacture of sticky, misfolded tau! This indicates that any anti-tau interventions may not be effective unless there is adequate fine-tuning of the GSK-3a activity upstream.

The narrowness of the optimal operating range complicates interventions aimed at GSK-3a. Turning GSK-3a's "volume" down too low is incompatible with life. High-decibel GSK-3a activity counterproductively cranks up rogue protein formation. Another tricky point of order is that GSK-3a is closely partnered to a fussy protein called "Notch." Tickle Notch production the wrong way, and animal models of Alzheimer's die in the fetal stage of life or patients get skin cancer. Those kinds of adverse effects are deal-breakers.

Scientists have been hot on the trail of a GSK-3a blocker for decades, and they have only recently arrived at a stage where they can inhibit GSK without sacrificing the production of Notch. Lithium is an example of one candidate that did not pan out as an effective GSK-3a inhibitor, although it seemed to work in the petri dish. This work has only gone through the pre-clinical development, however, and it may be another 10 years before you can access it as a prescription drug.

Once we do find the right drug or protein to combat protein-opathy, there remains the challenge of how to deliver it to the brain regions that need it most. The blood–brain barrier is the equivalent of a barbed-wire fence erected to protect the brain from foreign agents, whether toxic substances or infectious particles. The downside of having this nearly impenetrable barbed wire around the brain can sometimes mean that the brain is trapped inside of that fence, locked away from agents that might help it to overcome internal disasters, such as proteinopathy. A nasal spray is one way of drifting the medication into the brain, bypassing the acidic stomach and the long journey through the circulatory system and across the blood–brain barrier.

Another delivery route is via the stem cell. Stem cells are, to a certain extent, programmable and can then be transplanted into more mature, already-developed tissues to assimilate and carry out their programs. One could engineer a stem cell to produce replacements for what the brain is missing in dementia. Or, we could use the stem cell as a Trojan horse to deliver agents that can combat rogue proteins, and specifically sharpshoot into the brain regions targeted by the dementia. Researchers are getting closer every year to developing this technology.

The ability to capitalize on stem cell transplantation is much less controversial than is the source of the stem cells. Researchers in Korea have been leading experiments to transplant stem cells from cows into humans, which avoids debates brought by those who assume all stem cells come from aborted fetuses. Investigators avoid the emotional controversy around stem cell research by referring to their work as "induced pluripotent stem cells," or iPSCs, for those who want to keep themselves up-to-date through Google searching.

Topping the Most Wanted list of rogue proteins has been beta-amyloid, a key player in Alzheimer's disease. In 2012, there were 30 anti-amyloid interventions under active testing and an order of magnitude fewer for anti-tau interventions. Amyloid has been more popular because the genetics have shown more links to beta-amyloid than to tau, the other major suspect in the proteinopathy of Alzheimer's disease.

One of the most highly anticipated anti-amyloid interventions under development in the last decade has been the vaccine. Among industrialized nations, mandatory vaccination to prevent epidemics of illness, especially among children, has become routine practice. When the results of testing the first vaccine against rogue amyloid were reported, I was happy to think we were going to have an intervention that the lay public could readily understand. Even those who do not believe in mandatory vaccinations for children can understand the biological mechanism by which a vaccine can help prevent illness. In the ideal scenario, each of us could get a one-time vaccine against the beta form of amyloid at any point up to mid-life; that would allow us to avoid Alzheimer's disease because our bodies would produce antibodies against amyloid to tag it for garbage disposal by the immune system!

Of course, that sounded like a pipe dream ... until in 1999 Dale Schenk presented the results of his experiments on mice that had been engineered to develop amyloid plaques over the course of their short lives. The slides showed amazing results. Essentially, there was a "Now you see it, now you don't" difference between mice doomed to plaque formation and their brethren who received the vaccine early in life. The excitement that followed his talk was palpable. Schenk was reporting the results of "pre-clinical trials," which use animal models of the disease as the experimental subjects. The next step, of course, was to test the vaccine in humans.

After non-human testing, subsequent clinical trials are labeled by phase: Phase I describes a safety trial that addresses the issue of whether the drug as formulated is tolerated by young, healthy humans (generally college student volunteers) who do not have the target disease. That first vaccine against Alzheimer's disease used in mice coasted through Phase I.

Phase II is the evidence you're looking for to find treatment for a loved one. If Phase II trial results are positive, that means that an initial group of patients with the disease has been able to tolerate the drug, and there is reason to expect that the drug will be further developed by the manufacturer for distribution to the public.

Phase III trials determine the efficacy of the drug at different doses. They can answer questions such as, "How many times should a person get the vaccine?" and "Where is the perfect balance between effective and safe?"

Phase IV trials give a longer view of what has happened to patients after the official approval of the drug, or may be seeking secondary indications (new types of dementia) that will respond to the drug after it was approved for use against one illness.

There was good news and there was bad news about the Phase II clinical trials of the vaccine against Alzheimer's disease. The good news was that patients who received the vaccine had fewer amyloid plaques in their brains at autopsy than would have been expected, given the duration of illness. The bad news was that a small proportion of study participants had a very strong immune reaction to receiving the vaccine, so strong that it caused seizures and irritation of the meninges, the outer membrane covering the brain. Ever since then, there has been a hot race to develop a different way to immunize against rogue amyloid. The latest attempts have been using what is called passive immunotherapy. The idea here is to provide the small antibodies to the patient, instead of exposing the body to the foreign body to trigger it to make its own antibodies against amyloid (which runs the risk of inciting an overreaction from the immune system). Neil Cashman of the University of British Columbia is working to develop antibody therapy that could control the prion activity that may underlie the spreading process of dementia within the brain.

What of tau, the other apparent Alzheimer's culprit? A transgenic rat has been created to test a vaccine made from truncated tau to address tauopathy. Early results show not only a decrease in the neurofibrillary tangles but also a delay in the progression of outward signs of brain disturbance. Otherwise, the main ways to get rid of tau would be (1) to interfere with its phosphorylation, the process that makes tau sticky and tangle-forming, or (2) to reinforce the microtubule structure of the neuron against the faulty tau building blocks being made by the patient's brain.

Paclitaxel, a drug used against breast cancer, shows anti-tau activity in a petri dish but is too difficult to get into the brain effectively. This may be just as well, as breast cancer survivors have complained about chronic vertigo and not feeling as cognitively sharp when they are taking paclitaxel. The lithium story has proceeded similarly: It showed anti-tau properties when in a petri dish yet was not so good in patients for that purpose. Patients taking lithium for bipolar affective disorder are already too aware of the most common side effects of this drug: tremor, lowering of thyroid hormone release, and acne. Instead, the focus has turned to a molecule structurally similar to lithium, called epithelone. Virginia Lee and John Trojanowski have been tracking down a silver bullet for tau from their stronghold at the University of Pennsylvania's Center for Neurodegenerative Research since 2002.

Regarding other types of dementia, we still await candidate agents to test. There are indications that drugs that have been used in psychiatric disorders may have additional uses to combat prion diseases. Creutzfeldt–Jakob disease is a prion disease, occurring rarely. If Alzheimer's disease does turn out to be a prion disease (the first evidence has been in a petri dish), perhaps the same treatment could be used for both, as well as for other dementias.

Going from pre-clinical through Phases I–III of drug testing is not only expensive but time-consuming, taking up to a decade in addition to the first decade it took to get through pre-clinical testing. One shortcut to making a drug available to patients is the open-label trial. Once a medication has already received approval from a drug regulation agency for one disease, the researcher can try the same drug in similar conditions, if he can propose a decent connection to the drug's mechanism of action.

Some clinicians skip even the open-label trial process—because the drug is at the pharmacy, already approved by Health Canada for another condition—and write a prescription for the drug. That practice is called "off-label" prescribing. Our reasoning is usually that the patient cannot wait for formal approvals, and the potential benefit outweighs the risk of side effects. Doctors should disclose when and why they are writing off-label prescriptions, because if something untoward results, they are liable. However, it should be noted that the overwhelming majority of prescriptions written for patients with dementia are off-label! That antidepressant that's intended to help reduce irritability does not carry an indication specifically "to address irritability in the context of Alzheimer's disease." It was originally indicated instead for depression or stabilization of a mood disorder, but the potential to reduce severe irritability that is keeping a patient and caregiver from enjoying a better quality of life may be worth a try.

When there's a new medication that might benefit a large number of my clinic patients, I try to organize an open-label trial, as opposed to writing off-label prescriptions, because it commits me to evaluating the efficacy of the drug in a uniform, more objective way. That way any observations I make about the drug's effectiveness can be applied usefully to other doctors' practices. An example of an open-label trial was our test of memantine, a drug originally approved for use in moderate-to-severe-stage Alzheimer's disease. We wanted to test whether it would also work for a different dementia—frontotemporal dementia.

William and Jenny were a Michigan couple who participated in the trial. William was keen to get his wife Jenny involved in the memantine study, even though it meant driving her to Toronto several times to participate. There were no other available drug trials for frontotemporal dementia in their region, and they understood that acting early is often more effective than waiting until the dementia has advanced. Our clinical drug trial (NCT 00594737 on www.clinicaltrials.gov) tested the effects of memantine on the appearance of the brain as it devours radioactive glucose. This type of imaging is called FDG-PET (for fluoro-deoxy-glucose positron emission tomography), and it can reveal telltale patterns of brain dysfunction. The more advanced the dementia, the less glucose the brain absorbs; the lighted areas on the FDG-PET provide a map to the most intact brain regions. The diminishing glucose signal is not specific to a disease, but the pattern of lowered signal across brain regions can be specific to some dementias.

William and Jenny arrived in Toronto hopeful. I carefully went through the informed consent with them, emphasizing several times that the use of memantine in this context was experimental. To justify this type of study ethically, the scientists need to acknowledge that we *don't* know and can't promise that the drug will work. It states clearly on the form that "the participant may not directly benefit from volunteering for this study." I especially appreciated that William and Jenny were willing to take this risk, even if they had to travel at their own expense to complete the study. They and so many of our patients graciously contribute the knowledge gained from such studies to others with dementia, even if the drug ultimately does not work for the participant.

Jenny, who'd started with loss of speech, showed less hot glucose to light up her left hemisphere language brain regions. We looked for those dark regions to become brighter after use of the drug in Jenny and in 16 other participants with frontotemporal dementia. The first pre-drug PET scan helped us to confirm diagnoses, and the second PET scan told us if anything had changed during the first two months of taking the medication. When they drove into town for the second PET scan, they let me know that after I'd last seen them, Immigration had detained Jenny at the Canada–U.S. border because she had retained enough radioactivity from the baseline PET to set off the metal detector! I made sure to write them a letter to carry with them explaining the issue. Patients typically are no longer "hot" by bedtime on the day of their FDG-PET scans, but William and

Jenny were saving on their cost of study participation by driving home directly after the PET scan.

More surprisingly, they reported that Jenny had improved with the medication, despite the short time since its start. Medications approved for Alzheimer's disease have a six-month interval over which to prove themselves worthy; Jenny had been taking memantine for just two months. Jenny reported, "I feel like I've gotten my life back."

Before running out to buy memantine, however, please consider that this is just one person giving her subjective comment on the study drug. She was one of several who wished to continue taking the medication after the study formally ended, and she is probably the person who placed the most stock in its effect. Sadly, the perceived benefit did not last, and not many other participants with frontotemporal dementia got as much out of taking the medication. One other participant in my study claimed he felt better immediately after each brain scan (MRI and PET), so we don't know whether to interpret that as placebo effect or drug effect. That is why placebo-controlled studies are so important. Results from Jenny and the others in the memantine trial, taken as a group, showed that memantine is improving the FDG signal that has been lowered in patients with frontotemporal dementia, particularly in a brain circuit called the salience network. That was an exciting result, because this part of the brain seems most vulnerable to frontotemporal dementia TDP-43 build-up. But patients across the board did not announce that they were feeling sharper. I am intrigued.

It is hard to conduct research without conflicts of interest arising. Ethics review boards are convened to help protect subjects against these issues. If a pharmaceutical company has funded a large-scale Phase II clinical drug trial, the investigator can make upwards of $10,000 per subject enrolled and often more if the subject completes the study. This creates a need to ensure that the scientific method remains a higher priority than clinical trial program cash flow. Even if no money were to change hands, academic researchers' career promotions rely upon completing studies and publishing their results. It is more difficult to publish a negative study reporting that a drug was ineffective than a positive one, and this raises the temptation to fudge the data. The consequences of such deception can be disastrous, inciting false hope and causing the misappropriation of health care resources. Another pressure on researchers may be generated by their own institutions. Hospitals and other health care centers are very keen to promote their work as groundbreaking and cutting edge, to attract donors. In some cases, the preference of the donor or sponsoring agency may drive the decisions about which drug will be tested or on which type of patient.

Sometimes the agency that funded the study has control over whether the results are made public. The movie *Thank You for Smoking* illustrates an extreme example of the American tobacco industry creating its own research institute to control the public's understanding of the ill effects of smoking.

There is a large gray zone between the economic reality of conducting research and what's best for the stakeholders. There's high financial risk to develop and test these agents, costing about one billion dollars to bring one drug to market. But given the soaring Boomer population, the gain would be worth it. At minimum, there should always be transparency as to what the potential conflicts of interest are. The stakeholders include the organizations supporting the lab, not just the patients affected by disease. I was pleased to note the balanced press release about the discovery of a new drug for Alzheimer's, bexarotene. It featured this disclaimer from principal investigator Gary Landreth at Case Western: "I want to say as loudly and clearly as possible that this was a study in mice, not in humans. We've fixed Alzheimer's in mice lots of times [without later seeing the same results in humans], so we need to move forward expeditiously but cautiously."

Finding treatment for dementia requires finding several treatments that would be used according to a patient's stage of illness: at genetic risk but not manifesting signs; already showing mild signs; halfway through cognitive losses; and requiring reversal of an end stage. Although there is no proven cure on the pharmacist's shelf currently, we have some exciting leads on how to muzzle the hosts (potentially prions) of the unwanted destructive party. We also have a better understanding of who the bouncers protecting the brain are (e.g., GSK-3a, microRNAs, and chaperone proteins), and we need to know how to sustain their function late into life. We may eventually develop a way to activate the immune system so that it can clear away abnormal proteins (vaccine). We will find true solutions only after we can come to a very comprehensive view of the complexity that allows dementia to start and to accelerate.

14

LOOKING TOWARD THE HORIZON OF THIS FIELD

There are no great limits to growth because there are no limits of human intelligence, imagination, and wonder.

—FORMER U.S. PRESIDENT RONALD REAGAN,
AND THE WORLD'S MOST FAMOUS ALZHEIMER' S DISEASE PATIENT

I like to think the complexity of searching for treatment for dementia will eventually have a happy ending. Looking back over medical history, we have seen how illness causes fear, avoidance, and isolation. We have also seen how the kindness and openness of people who want to end that suffering opens doors to treatment and healing. With my Hawai'ian roots, I turn for inspiration to the desolate story of the exile of patients with Hansen's disease (also known as leprosy) to the island of Moloka'i. The Moloka'i story began with "There's no cure," but its eventual resolution gives me hope that there is a happy ending for dementia care ahead. Persistent compassion and equanimity eventually led to triumph over a slow but relentless fatal illness.

The exile of those diagnosed and misdiagnosed with Hansen's disease was in full swing through Ah Quan's life. She never spoke of it to me directly, but her generation had spoken enough about it in their own households to instill a sense of dread in my parents, which remains to this day. They recoiled a bit when I mentioned I was reading books on the subject.

I feel my family has a personal connection to the Moloka'i story, because the first of the missionary Judd family sailed to Hawai'i on the same boat from New England as Reverend Jonathan Green, and the Green family raised Ah Quan. Three generations of Judds played significant roles in the leper settlement on Moloka'i. First, Dr. Gerrit P. Judd made the initial diagnoses of Hansen's disease in people from each of the Islands. His handwritten notes report a biblical connection, contagion among the poor, and that the government (goaded on by his son) had tried to establish quarantine. He wrote, "This is apparently a scourge sent from God upon those who neglect the proprieties of life. It is often hereditary owing to fault of one or both parents."

Dr. Judd's son Albert, the chief justice of the Hawai'ian Supreme Court, had a more commercial than medical interest in this twentieth-century "plague" and used his influence with the last monarchs to arrange for the exile of leprosy patients to Moloka'i, under the ruse that they were being sent to a special hospital. United States territory status was heavily supported by pineapple and sugarcane plantation owners who had come from New England to capitalize on this business opportunity. Some of them had come as missionaries, but saw the value of the land and then were able to get away with cheaper labor costs in a U.S. territory than in a U.S. state. It was going to be very bad for business if food products coming from "diseased" ground underwent embargo. Albert himself explained, "Leprosy makes you a pariah, someone who is cast out and mustn't touch anyone."

Some Hawai'ians had to disavow their own affected family members in order to save family-sustaining businesses. Poor, immigrant Asian-Pacific Islanders were not the only people exiled to desolate, inescapable Moloka'i. Eventually, there were members from all levels of socioeconomic status, including Hawai'ian royalty, shipped away from their homes to Moloka'i.

Where was equanimity? Where was compassion? Father Damien was not the only person who volunteered to help the patients on Moloka'i, although he is probably the most famous one. It was, of all people, Dr. Judd's grandson, Lawrence McCully Judd, the seventh territorial governor of Hawai'i, who ultimately ensured that antibiotic treatment was made available to patients as soon as it was developed in Louisiana. Prior to that, he had fought for more humane conditions and for reuniting patients with their families. Lawrence had grown up just a few doors down from where Ah Quan lived with the Green family.

The Moloka'i story interweaves numerous compassionate acts that accumulated over time; a community formed from a core of people quarantined in a forbidding environment, where children were later born and educated. The leper settlement, Kalaupapa, was so inaccessible that the exiles were forced to swim from the boat onto the rocky shores of West Moloka'i. Many never made it to Kalaupapa. By 1969, it was no longer illegal to remain in your own home while receiving treatment for Hansen's disease, and the communities of Kalaupapa and neighboring Kalawao were approved to be commemorated as historical places respecting the patients who had suffered.

At the beginning of exile to Moloka'i, people were still trying to wrap their minds around the concept of germs, let alone the development of an antibiotic. While patients with dementia have not been deemed contagious, there is a parallel of stigmatization associated with the illness, and there is a dire need for a scientific approach to bridge the huge gap in knowledge about this disease. The economic consequences of the epidemic, and the importance of kindness and compassion for the patients as people with an illness, apply to dementing illness. Imagine if we were to pack anyone with a cancer diagnosis off to a remote island! Ah Quan was 53 when Hawai'i became the fiftieth state of the United States. People were still being exiled to Moloka'i 10 years into Hawai'i's statehood.

Patients with dementia sometimes express fear of exile to nursing homes. I wonder how much our aversion to people aging *un*successfully encourages the elderly to move to retirement homes, assisted-living facilities, or nursing homes. Undeniably, physically frail older adults or highly agitated patients with dementia are at much higher risk of coming to harm if they are living without help in their own homes. But the solution that reflects more equanimity may be to integrate them into vibrant, multigenerational community life, instead of placing them among other unhealthy elderly people with poor prognoses. The story of Moloka'i reinforces how, in the absence of a quicker fix, kindness and compassion are vital to keeping life moving in a positive direction. Instead of exile to Moloka'i constituting a death or prison sentence, survivors with Hansen's disease were able to build a sense of integration into a community, one that lived with the disfigurement and dying, along with celebrating the lives of children born there without Hansen's disease, for whom they could imagine a better life.

When I asked Grandpa how he endured his first year without Grandma, he did not go into detailed memories of what he missed most about her. To him her absence was so overwhelming that it defied description. He alternated between answers, "We were together for 71 years," and "It's very hard without her."

Ah Quan navigated the neighborhood with Grandpa patiently at her elbow, warning of obstacles they encountered on their strolls to the library or store. Even though she had Alzheimer's, it was an atypical form, allowing her to recall with startling clarity friends' and neighbors' family histories. She could also recount in dizzying detail the latest large-print romance novel; she never tired of the bodice-ripper formula.

Ah Quan did not awaken after her hemorrhagic stroke. I can still see the white amorphous blob on her CT scan as I held it up to the light, standing at her bedside with her doctor in the aloha shirt. I think of this whenever I review brain scans on patients who have had intracranial bleeds. I grade them as appearing larger than, smaller than, or much like Grandma's. And each time I see those scans, I am grateful that, despite the brain injury, Grandma looked so perfectly peaceful in bed, as if she could pop out of her afternoon nap to enjoy a few of her individually waxed paper–wrapped Dream Cookies (it keeps them crispy and whole, even after trans-Pacific shipping!) with a glass of milk.

Marjorie, my patient who began to have symptoms of Alzheimer's disease in her late forties, and her husband, Mark, will not have had the same opportunity to age together gracefully. It is hard to know whether to wish for them a quick course of illness, as so often happens with early-onset cases, or a long drift away from the life that they have known with their children. Most recently, Marjorie has delighted in a newfound activity, drawing abstracted nature. I love the smile on her face as she attempts to explain what she likes most about each piece. I can't help but smile when I recall it. Given that we don't have much control over the situation, it is of some comfort to think in terms of the four intentions: However long Marjorie has the disease, we hope that she will always feel safe, that she will always feel loved, that each day will bring some joy, and that she will be physically comfortable.

The closest I've ever come to feeling the functional losses in a family member with dementia was when my own godparents attended an appointment at my UCLA clinic. My parents, while not officially subscribing to any one organized religion, had nevertheless wanted to make sure that someone would take care of my brother and me in case something untimely were to befall them. Our next-door neighbors, Max and Annie, were perfect candidates.

As a lawyer, Max could see to any estate proceedings. They had no children of their own, and living next door, they might be able to oversee us in our own home in the event that we were orphaned. Max and Annie were regular fixtures of my youth, waving and exchanging news of the day when we walked past their house, curious about how school was going for us, pleased when success came our way. Annie gave me my first exposure to a New York Jewish accent and her style of dress reminded me of Jackie O.

Only 16 years after I had left home for college, Max was

wheeling Annie into my clinic to become my patient, and neither of them recognized me, even after I described how we knew each other. My ego couldn't understand why these beloved neighbors didn't know to embrace me. But they were both safe, happy, and still obviously, tenderly loving each other. They were not in good health, but they were making sure to seek medical help. I had to let go of the roles they had played in my life to be able to give them accepting, kind care. Did it matter if they perceived it as coming from an interested stranger?

As I progress in age and my work, I will continue to look out for ways to tip the scales in my own favor, away from developing dementia. While the healthiest diet will be a daily challenge, keeping engaged with those around me and keeping engaged physically will happen fairly naturally, unless unforeseen illness or injury intervene. I can peek ahead quantitatively with a predictive formula for 20-year risk of dementia (see Appendix 3).

Whether you believe yourself or a loved one to be at high risk of getting dementia, the common assumption is that there will be a vast loss. North American adults spend most of their life creating an identity based on what they do for a living, how good they are at parenting, or how successful they are at creating a home and lifestyle. These attributes definitely change with dementia, regardless of what type has struck. In academics and most of industrialized life, the more one can multitask and the more one can produce, the greater one's perceived worth. But what, then, can life with dementia mean? Certainly the person who can no longer run an office should not be considered worthless. How do we reconcile that accidental stillness?

With every day of clinic, I learn from my patients and their families that life with cognitive impairment or dementia doesn't have to be devoid of quality. This is valuable dharma! Facing a life that is changing due to dementia often brings on opportunities for practicing loving kindness, joy, equanimity, and compassion. It is best to remain open to the good that can come with any changes.

DO-IT-YOURSELF—BELIEVING THE NEWSPAPER HEADLINES

If I could wave my magic wand, I would imbue each caregiver with the ability to sort critically through the information on dementia "breakthroughs" available on the internet. Although they are reading with some caution, caregivers forward all sorts of cure claims they find on the internet to me for an opinion. Some of this spurious material even makes its way as links onto otherwise trustworthy websites.

Here are some general rules of thumb you can use to evaluate whether the information is valid. If the article is about diagnostic testing, you'd like to see:

- validation of the test between people who have the illness confirmed by autopsy and an age-matched sample without the illness
- validation among participants who resemble your demographics (age, sex, race, ethnicity) and risk for dementia (presence or absence of family history)

- availability of the test to the general public (It may be exciting and promising, but where is it being conducted and what does it cost? New technology typically comes at a price and is not necessarily covered by your health insurance.)

If the article is about a new "breakthrough" treatment, it should explain:

- Were the participants included in the study affected by the target illness? Was the diagnosis made within the same guidelines that your doctor is using for you? There is a difference to you in results from a study conducted on patients *at risk* for a disease versus patients already diagnosed with the disease. Both types of studies may be valid, but the applicability of the results to you may differ. My patient Mimi recounts on every visit the findings of a *Reader's Digest* article in which a patient with Alzheimer's disease had a curative surgery. She insists she wants "someone to go in there [knocking on her head] and fiddle around, to bring back aaaaaall my memories." But even if the surgical result had been replicated in a decent number of Alzheimer's patients (it hasn't), Mimi doesn't understand that she does not have Alzheimer's disease. The article doesn't pertain to her.
- Is there a good rationale behind the use of the test drug? Researchers try to use logical means against the target illness—if we can't justify that the intervention acts on something with a known association to the disease mechanism (e.g., the abnormal protein, or a biochemical

process known to be deranged in the dementia), you'd need to be sure the study was soundly designed before you take much meaning from the study. Sometimes the rationale is based on observation; the curcumin trials arose from the observation that those who have an East Indian diet with a large amount of curcumin were at lower risk than others internationally for Alzheimer's disease. This led to a diet intervention trial and simultaneous bench studies checking the effects of curcumin on phosphorylated (sticky) tau.

- Was the study designed to test the drug against a placebo or another drug considered the current standard? The FDA and other public health drug agencies typically will not approve the drug unless it has shown clear superiority over a placebo or at least equivalence against another drug already available. If the drug is not approved by a drug regulatory agency, it will not be made available at the pharmacy.

- Were the outcomes of all the enrolled participants detailed? Sometimes the study is positive only for a small segment of the population and the other participants dropped out before the study ended, which skews the final statistical analysis. It's important to know who dropped out in case you more closely match that group than you do the study-completers.

- If there were a lot of study dropouts, did the investigators calculate the results by bringing the last observation forward? This is the authors' way of acknowledging that there were some holdups in the study for participants.

- Sometimes participants leave a study early because

they are experiencing adverse effects. What were the
side effects of the drug reported in the study? Are
they life-threatening? Did they occur with the same
frequency in the placebo group? Even if there is a
high risk of a few side effects, the benefit of the drug
may outweigh the risk in individual decision-making.
The relative economics of pharmaceutical drug
decision-making is a new science unto itself. The
fact that most dementias occur in elderly persons
who are at high risk of mortality due to age alone
can shift the decision-making algorithm for some
families.

- Is this article aimed at caregivers seeking affordable
treatment, or at venture capitalists looking to invest
in a drug that will sell well? The time from the end
of Phase I to the end of Phase III when the drug
can be widely accessible with a prescription can run
10–15 years minimum. When the newspaper headline
proclaims, "Breakthrough!," check to see if they're
talking about a pre-clinical, Phase I, or Phase III result.
A breakthrough announcement in the newspaper may
predate a prescription drug on your pharmacist's shelf
by 20 years.

- There's a difference between "statistically significant"
and "clinically significant." If you can afford to enroll
thousands of patients in a clinical trial, that number can
influence the statistics to highlight a very small difference that would not be just a chance finding. That is a
statistically significant difference. If my experimental
intervention were to wave hello to each patient every

morning in passing, and 1800 of the 2000 patients
showed a change in blood pressure from 170/85 to
165/85, the investigators could report a statistically
significant reduction in blood pressure (it did go down!)
from a "therapeutic wave." This amount of change in
blood pressure doesn't make much of a difference in life
outcomes such as stroke, heart attack, or sudden death.
This finding therefore wouldn't necessarily be *clinically*
significant. The most responsible of investigators would
choose a clinically significant amount of change (e.g., a
larger drop from 170 to 140 in systolic blood pressure)
before performing the study, then would report trans-
parently that they found only statistically significant
change at a level below clinical significance when they
published the results. A responsible scientific journal's
peer reviewers would insist that the results be stated in
this balanced way.

- Is the newspaper or a health website the only place
  where the results have been published? If so, peer
  reviewers at a reputable journal may not have agreed
  with the design, results, or phrasing of the report from
  the study.

- "What is the drug?" is important, but emerging work
  is also proving that *"When is the drug useful?"* is just
  as important. Consider the complexity of estrogen
  supplementation, for instance. We are still at the stage
  of discovering which abnormal protein collections are
  key to target with treatment first. Although Alzheimer's
  disease patients have abnormal tau and amyloid, it is not
  clear which target should be the priority, and the answer

may differ depending upon the age of the patient or level of cognitive impairment already in place.

- Whether it's a drug or a lifestyle intervention, the same questions above should be applied to the information. There are some suggestions that will seem like "common sense," such as, more exercise is better for you, but this may not be applicable to a patient with terrible arthritic pain on walking, or it may have greater impact at a different time of the lifespan than the one you're now in.

Newspaper articles often bear word limits and cannot express all these details. They will tell whether the study was an open-label drug study (implying no placebo arm) or placebo-controlled. To answer the critique questions, you may have to go to the original articles themselves, which are often available online through a hospital or university library. To get into print, studies must detail all of these parameters. Peer reviewers demand it. When in doubt, ask your doctor to help you interpret the applicability of the new findings to you specifically. It's what we are trained to do.

APPENDIX 2

DO-IT-YOURSELF—
VOLUNTEERING
FOR THE RESEARCH
THAT'S RIGHT FOR YOU

Whether you have dementia, think you'll get it, or feel like you will live on as a healthy control, we need you to participate in research! The ultimate is to allow a brain autopsy. Have you ever considered what happens when you "donate your body to science"? I highly recommend Mary Roach's book, *Stiff*, as a very reader-friendly report on what happens to bodies after death. Roach is a curious journalist, and her book illustrates that the squeamishness factor is the same whether a body decomposes or is cremated or is studied by a scientist. If you agree to brain autopsy, most centers will endeavor to have the rest of your body returned and available for viewing within 24 hours, if that is part of your family's request. Once we have removed the brain from the skull, part of the brain is frozen and the rest is fixed in formalin so that immunostains can be done on small slices to identify which abnormal proteins you might have harbored and where.

To locate clinical trials for your loved one, I always recommend www.clinicaltrials.gov. The entries onto this government-sponsored website are vetted to a small extent, in that proof of an ethics review board approval is required for all studies listed. However, some of the entries may be outdated (e.g., the study stopped recruiting a year ago) or the ethics review board that approved the study may not have the same high standards as others. As you pursue participation in a study, be VERY suspicious if:

- there is no mechanism for someone to answer your questions about the study (and there is NO such thing as a stupid question)
- you have not been informed equally well about benefits and risks of participating
- there are penalties for withdrawing from the study
- the patient with dementia can give consent in the absence of someone holding power of attorney

It is important to ask if you must stop medications the patient is already taking in order to participate. Depending upon whether you and your doctor think those medications are actively benefiting the patient, having to stop them for the study may be a deal-breaker.

Rights of the participant in a study should be stated on the informed consent form. These include:

- a written explanation of all study procedures, purposes, risks, and benefits
- the opportunity to ask questions and to feel that all questions have been answered satisfactorily before consenting to the study

- ample time to consider the risks and benefits before consenting to the study
- the ability to withdraw at any point in the study without penalties or adverse consequences to the patient's clinical care
- assurance of confidentiality

It is the researcher's responsibility to help patients and their families feel comfortable enough with the study procedures that they will be inclined to complete participation. We are disappointed if you have to leave the study early, but we know that your participation is voluntary. We do value your contribution of time and energy and especially your trust that we will act in *your* best interest in all events.

APPENDIX 3

HOW DO YOU MEASURE UP FOR RISK?

This applies to dementias of any type, not just Alzheimer's disease.

I'm sure this has not appeared as a *Cosmopolitan* magazine quiz yet, but Miia Kivipelto, an epidemiologist at the Karolinska Institutet, developed this risk scoring system in 2006. My total score places me into one of three risk profiles (low, intermediate, or high), based on mostly cardiovascular risk factors.

What is your age?
- Younger than 47; 0 points _____
- Between 47 and 53; 3 points _____
- Older than 53; 5 points (5) ✓_____

How much education do you have?
- More than 10 years; 0 points 0 ✓_____
- 7–9 years; 3 points _____
- Less than 7 years; 4 points _____

What is your sex?
- Female; 0 points   *0* ✓ _____
- Male; 1 point   _____

Yes, this does run counter to prior lore
that women are at higher risk
for Alzheimer's disease, the most
common form of dementia in the elderly.

What is your systolic blood pressure
(the first and larger number of
blood pressure)?
- Less than 140 mmHg; 0 points *0* ✓ _____
- 140 mmHg or greater; 2 points _____

Mine ranges from 90 to 100, which
contributes 0 out of 2 points possible for
this item to my score. There is no score
of 1 available for this item.

What is your body mass index (BMI)?
- Less than 30 kg/m²; 0 points _____
- Greater than 30 kg/m²; 1 point ✓ _____
                                 1

This measure is controversial. See Chapter 8,
"Think before You Eat." My BMI is 20.7,
which seems much lower than their
generous cutoff score of 30 kg/m², yet I
still have my muffin top!

What is your total cholesterol level?
- Less than 6.5 mmol/L; 0 points _____
- Greater than 6.5 mmol/L; 1 point ✓ _____

My total cholesterol was 5.3 mmol/L at last check. (Thank you, oh, Lord, for genetically allowing me bacon and cheese.)

How often are you physically active enough for 20–30 minutes per episode to cause sweat and breathlessness?
- At least twice a week; 0 points ✓ _____
- Less than twice a week; 1 point _____

I'm in the swimming pool twice a week, dancing twice a week, and in the gym maybe one other day per week.

What is your Apolipoprotein E genotype?
- No alleles; 0 points _____
- 1 or 2 alleles; 2 points _____

I haven't had my blood sent in for this test. But let's assume for the sake of this exercise that I do carry one APOE 4 allele.

Total score:
- **0–9: low risk** _____6_____
- **10–11: intermediate risk** _____
- **12–15: high risk** _____

My total score is 2. I'd rather have a score of zero, but anyone with a score of 0–9 fits into the same low-risk category. My risk of having dementia 20 years from today is 0.3%. This is good, since I have a lot of items on my to-do list to accomplish before I'm done with this life.

For those who have already lived through mid-life and are now in their seventies, there's a late-life checklist of weighted risk factors by Deborah Barnes, a psychiatrist at UC San Francisco. Disclaimer: Some of these points are controversial, as annotated.

- The closer you are to 80, the higher your score is.
- Poor current cognitive test performance implies that the horse is already out of the barn.
- BMI should be less than 18.5. (Huh?!?! That means I have to lose 16 pounds in the next 30 years. I can tell you right now, that's not going to happen. I'd have to run around inside the shower just to get wet. As written in Chapter 8, the general rule of thumb is to be neither too skinny nor too fat and then stay there.)
- One or two Apolipoprotein E4 alleles are present.
- MRI scan of the brain was abnormal. (Is there any indication to have an MRI scan just for the heck of it? Not yet.)
- There is evidence of atherosclerosis in carotid arteries.
- There is a history of coronary artery bypass graft surgery.
- Physical performance has slowed. (Although one might think slower walking due to arthritic changes shouldn't

count, but decreased activity may keep a person more isolated and less able to modulate blood and oxygen delivery to the brain.)

- There is a LACK of alcohol consumption. (The advice on this bullet item is to "drink WITHIN MODERATION.")

Your score on this late-life dementia risk index will predict what life will be like six years from now. You may enjoy six times the reduction of dementia risk relative to the rest of the pack, if you're a low-scorer. Low-scorers carry only a 4% risk of developing dementia, while moderate-scorers have a 23% risk of developing dementia before the next decade passes. But wait, there's more: If you're a high-scorer, look out, because your risk is not just 46%; it's jumped to **56%**. A moderate-scorer might delude himself that he can hide in the odds and not be the one out of four peers who will have dementia, but fifty-fifty odds (for the high-scorers) are almost forbidding. The factors in this list for older individuals are definitely related to the factors in the list for mid-life, so the take-home point is to study up on how to keep or earn membership in the low-scoring group posthaste.

NOTES

INTRODUCTION: LIFE LESSONS FROM THE MEMORY CLINIC
For more on Ah Quan's particular type of Alzheimer's disease:
Viswanathan, A., and S. M. Greenberg. "Cerebral Amyloid Angiopathy
  in the Elderly." *Annals of Neurology* 70, no. 6 (2011): 871–80.

**For more on loving kindness, I recommend just about anything by Sharon*
Salzberg. www.sharonsalzberg.com. I listen to her dharma talks through
www.dharmaseed.org when I'm feeling a little overwhelmed by life.
The downloads are free, but please do consider contributing what you
can to the cause. Dharma talks by Phillip Moffit (see Chapter 8) are
also available through Dharmaseed.

For my former instructor's tips on the socialization involved in
becoming a physician:
Coombs, Robert. *Surviving Medical School.* Sage Publications, Inc.,
  1998.

CHAPTER 2

For more on the types of abnormal proteins associated with different dementias:

Ito, D., and N. Suzuki. "Conjoint Pathologic Cascades Mediated by ALS/FTLD-U Linked RNA-Binding Proteins TDP-43 and FUS." *Neurology* 77, no. 17 (2011): 1636–43.

CHAPTER 3

For more about cognitive reserve:

Borroni, B., et al. "Revisiting Brain Reserve Hypothesis in Fronto-temporal Dementia: Evidence from a Brain Perfusion Study." *Dementia and Geriatric Cognitive Disorders* 28, no. 2 (2009): 130–5.

Pavlik, V. N., R. S. Doody, P. J. Massman, and W. Chan. "Influence of Premorbid IQ and Education on Progression of Alzheimer's Disease." *Dementia and Geriatric Cognitive Disorders* 22, no. 4 (2006): 367–77.

Roe, C. M., M. A. Mintun, G. D'Angelo, C. Xiong, E. A. Grant, and J. C. Morris. "Alzheimer Disease and Cognitive Reserve: Variation of Education Effect with Carbon 11-Labeled Pittsburgh Compound B Uptake." *Archives of Neurology* 65, no. 11 (2008): 1467–71.

Roe, C. M., C. Xiong, J. P. Miller, and J. C. Morris. "Education and Alzheimer Disease without Dementia: Support for the Cognitive Reserve Hypothesis." *Neurology* 68, no. 3 (2007): 223–8.

Satz, P. "Brain Reserve Capacity on Symptom Onset after Brain Injury: A Formulation." *Proceedings of the Royal Society London* 58 (1965): 295–300.

Scarmeas, N., and Y. Stern. "Cognitive Reserve and Lifestyle." *Journal of Clinical and Experimental Neuropsychology* 25, no. 5 (2003): 625–33.

Stern, Y. "Cognitive Reserve." *Neuropsychologia* 47, no. 10 (2009): 2015–28.

Stern, Y., B. Gurland, T. K. Tatemichi, M. X. Tang, D. Wilder, and R. Mayeux. "Influence of Education and Occupation on the Incidence of Alzheimer's Disease." *Journal of the American Medical Association* 271, no. 13 (1994): 1004–10.

Valenzuela, M.J. "Brain Reserve and Dementia: A Systematic Review." *Psychological Medicine* 36 (2006): 441–54.

Yaffe, K., et al. "Association of Plasma Beta-Amyloid Level and Cognitive Reserve with Subsequent Cognitive Decline." *Journal of the American Medical Association* 305, no. 3 (2011): 261–6.

For more information about missionaries in Hawai'i: www.missionhouses.org

For more about the different types of intelligence: Gladwell, Malcolm. *Outliers.* Little, Brown and Company, 2008.

For a description of the Nun Study:

Snowdon, D. A., S. J. Kemper, J. A. Mortimer, L. H. Greiner, D. R. Wekstein, and W. R. Markesbery. "Linguistic Ability in Early Life and Cognitive Function and Alzheimer's Disease in Late Life. Findings from the Nun Study." *Journal of the American Medical Association* 275, no. 7 (1996): 528–32.

CHAPTER 4

For more information about Dr. Pawan Sinha's work in India: web.mit.edu/bcs/sinha/prakash.html and www.nei.nih.gov/news/science advances/discovery/project_prakash.asp.

For more information about leisure activities and late-life cognitive training:

Akbaraly, T. N., et al. "Leisure Activities and the Risk of Dementia in the Elderly: Results from the Three-City Study." *Neurology* 73, no. 11 (2009): 854–61.

Hall, C. B., R. B. Lipton, M. Sliwinski, M. J. Katz, C. A. Derby, and J. Verghese. "Cognitive Activities Delay Onset of Memory Decline in Persons Who Develop Dementia." *Neurology* 73, no. 5 (2009): 356–61.

Hatch, S. L., et al. "The Continuing Benefits of Education: Adult Education and Midlife Cognitive Ability in the British 1946 Birth Cohort." *Journal of Gerontology Series B: Psychological Sciences and Social Sciences* 62, no. 6 (2007): S404–414.

Lindstrom, H. A., et al. "The Relationships between Television Viewing in Midlife and the Development of Alzheimer's Disease in a Case-Control Study." *Brain and Cognition* 58, no. 2 (2005): 157–65.

Pillai, J. A., C. B. Hall, D. W. Dickson, H. Buschke, R. B. Lipton, and J. Verghese. "Association of Crossword Puzzle Participation with Memory Decline in Persons Who Develop Dementia." *Journal of International Neuropsychology Society* 17, no. 6 (2011): 1006–13.

Willis, S. L., et al. "Long-Term Effects of Cognitive Training on Everyday Functional Outcomes in Older Adults." *Journal of the American Medical Association* 296, no. 23 (2006): 2805–14.

CHAPTER 5

For websites to look up genome project updates:

Alzheimer Research Forum. www.alzgene.org

Oak Ridge National. www.ornl.gov/sci/techresources/Human_Genome/faq/snps.shtml

For more details about genetic risk factors:

Dartigues, J. F., and C. Feart. "Risk Factors for Alzheimer Disease: Aging Beyond Age?" *Neurology* 77, no. 3 (2011): 206–7.

Lock, M., et al. "Susceptibility Genes and the Question of Embodied Identity." *Medical Anthropology Quarterly* 21, no. 3 (2007): 256–76.

For an overview of Richard Mayeux's work, which is too prolific to include all citations: www.cumc.columbia.edu/dept/sergievsky/fs/mayeux.html

CHAPTER 6

For more detailson childbearing and Alzheimer's disease risk:

White, J. A., M. McGue, and L. L. Heston. "Fertility and Parental Age in Alzheimer Disease." *Journal of Gerontology* 41, no. 1 (1986): 40–43.

Chapter 7

**I love that someone of this calibre came forward to bust the myth that women can or should try to "do it all."* See Anne-Marie Slaughter's cover story, "Why Women Still Can't Have It All," *The Atlantic* 2012: July/ August issue.

For caregiver support organizations:

Alzheimer's Association. www.alz.org

Alzheimer Society of Canada. www.alzheimer.ca

The Association for Frontotemporal Degeneration. www.theaftd.org

Lewy Body Dementia Association. www.lewybodydementia.org

There are many networks working with Alzheimer's associations to disseminate information or publicize educational events. I refer people regularly to the Toronto Dementia Network (www.dementiatoronto. org) and to the Canadian Dementia Knowledge Translation Network (www.lifeandminds.ca).

For caregivers who want to know more about ambiguous loss and the efficacy of managing it:

Boss, P. *Ambiguous Loss: Learning to Live with Unresolved Grief.* Boston: Harvard University Press, 2000.

Boss, P. *Loss, Trauma, and Resilience: Therapeutic Work with Ambiguous Loss.* W. W. Norton, 2006.

Olazaran J., et al. "Nonpharmacological Therapies in Alzheimer's Disease: A Systematic Review of Efficacy." *Dementia and Geriatric Cognitive Disorders* 30 (2010): 161–178.

**For a wonderful perspective on caregiver attitude akin to that demonstrated by Brian for Wendy, see Bell, V. and D. Troxel. *A Dignified Life, Revised and Expanded: The Best Friends™ Approach to Alzheimer's Care: A Guide for Care Partners.* HCI, 2012. I still distribute the list of "What Is a Best Friend?" (e.g., "friends laugh together often") to almost all caregivers in my clinic.*

Gail Elliot is a consultant who can help caregivers take a creative and helpful approach to their interactions with patients who have dementia: www.dementiability.com

Similarly, Cameron Camp helps teach how to have a good visit with someone who has dementia. See his website for the Center for Applied Research in Dementia: cen4ard.com

For statistics on the burden of caregiving:

Hollander, M. J., G. Liu, and N. L. Chappell. "Who Cares and How Much? The Imputed Economic Contribution to the Canadian Healthcare System of Middle-Aged and Older Unpaid Caregivers Providing Care to the Elderly." *Healthcare Quarterly* 12 (2009): 42–49.

Risk Analytica. *Rising Tide: Impact of Dementia on Canadian Society*, 2009. www.alzheimer.ca/en/Get-involved/Raise-your-voice/Rising-Tide/Rising-tide-summary

For more on the contribution of stress to Alzheimer's disease:

Holmes, C., C. Cunningham, E. Zotova, D. Culliford, and V. H. Perry. "Proinflammatory Cytokines, Sickness Behavior, and Alzheimer Disease." *Neurology* 77, no. 3 (2011): 212–218.

Holtzheimer, P. E., and H. S. Mayberg. "Stuck in a Rut: Rethinking Depression and Its Treatment." *Trends in Neuroscience* 34, no. 1 (2011): 1–9.

Pruessner, J. C., et al. "Self-Esteem, Locus of Control, Hippocampal Volume, and Cortisol Regulation in Young and Old Adulthood." *Neuroimage* 28 (2005): 815–26.

Sapolsky, R. *A Primate's Memoir*. Scribner, 2002.

For more on the benefits of an open mind and heart:
Suzuki, S., and D. Chadwick. *Zen Mind, Beginner's Mind*. Shambhala, 2011.

For an example of Bobby McFerrin's improvisational singing for amateur dancers in the audience, see www.youtube.com/watch?v=VW8sfNGzQeM

CHAPTER 8
**Highly recommended for good writing and knowledgeable balance:*
Greenberg, P. *Four Fish*. Penguin Press HC, 2010.

**In addition to* In Defense of Food, *Michael Pollan has a book out for those who have less time for reading. I glanced through this at the airport and still repeat some of the simply stated rules, such as considering meat as a flavoring for your meal, not the main attraction.* Pollan, M. *Food Rules: An Eater's Manual*. Penguin Books, 2012.

For Dr. Joe Schwarcz's constantly updated comments on the latest "toxin," see: oss.mcgill.ca/index.php or www.mcgill.ca/oss/blog

For more info on or by Phillip Moffit, see www.lifebalanceinstitute.com/phillip-moffitt

For more on obesity or diet:
Biggs, M. L., et al. "Association between Adiposity in Midlife and Older Age and Risk of Diabetes in Older Adults." *Journal of the American Medical Association* 303, no. 24 (2010): 2504–12.
Hughes, T. F., et al. "Midlife Fruit and Vegetable Consumption and Risk of Dementia in Later Life in Swedish Twins." *American Journal of Geriatric Psychiatry* 18, no. 5 (2010): 413–20.

Luchsinger, J. A., D. Cheng, M. X. Tang, N. Schupf, and R. Mayeux. "Central Obesity in the Elderly Is Related to Late-Onset Alzheimer Disease." *Alzheimer Disease and Associated Disorders* (2011).

Sano, M., et al. "A Controlled Trial of Selegiline, Alpha-Tocopherol, or Both as Treatment for Alzheimer's Disease. The Alzheimer's Disease Cooperative Study." *New England Journal of Medicine* 336, no. 17 (1997): 1216–22.

Soreca, I., et al. "Gain in Adiposity across 15 Years Is Associated with Reduced Gray Matter Volume in Healthy Women." *Psychosomatic Medicine* 71, no. 5 (2009): 485–90.

Wang, J., et al. "Moderate Consumption of Cabernet Sauvignon Attenuates Abeta Neuropathology in a Mouse Model of Alzheimer's Disease." *Federation of American Societies for Experimental Biology Journal* 20, no. 13 (2006): 2313–20.

For evidence on how important eating is in Asian culture:

Jones, R., T. W. Chow, and M. Gatz. "Asian Americans and Alzheimer's Disease: Assimilation, Culture, and Beliefs." *Journal of Aging Studies* 20 (2006): 11–25.

Pang, F. C., et al. "Effect of Neuropsychiatric Symptoms of Alzheimer's Disease on Chinese and American Caregivers." *International Journal of Geriatric Psychiatry* 17, no. 1 (2002): 29–34.

CHAPTER 9

For details on the impact of exercise on dementia risk:

Baker, L. D., et al. "Effects of Aerobic Exercise on Mild Cognitive Impairment: A Controlled Trial." *Archives of Neurology* 67, no. 1 (2010): 71–9.

Berchtold, N. C., et al. "Exercise Primes a Molecular Memory for Brain-Derived Neurotrophic Factor Protein Induction in the Rat Hippocampus." *Neuroscience* 133, no. 3 (2005): 853–61.

Buchman A. S., et al. "Total Daily Physical Activity and the Risk of AD and Cognitive Decline in Older Adults." *Neurology* 78, no. 17 (2012): 1323–9.

Langlois, F., T. T. Vu, K. Chassé, G. Dupuis, M. J. Kergoat, and L. Bherer. "The Benefits of Physical Exercise Training on Cognition and Quality of Life in Frail Older Adults." *Journal of Gerontology: Psychological Sciences*, 2012. [Epub ahead of print].

Larson, E. B., et al. "Exercise Is Associated with Reduced Risk for Incident Dementia Among Persons 65 Years of Age and Older." *Annals of Internal Medicine* 144, no. 2 (2006): 73–81.

Maesako, M., et al. "Exercise Is More Effective than Diet Control in Preventing High Fat Diet-Induced Beta-Amyloid Deposition and Memory Deficit in Amyloid Precursor Protein Transgenic Mice." *Journal of Biological Chemistry* 287, no. 27 (2012): 23024–33.

Mortimer, J. A., et al. "Changes in Brain Volume and Cognition in a Randomized Trial of Exercise and Social Interaction in a Community-Based Sample of Non-Demented Chinese Elders." *Journal of Alzheimer's Disease* 30, no. 4 (2012): 757–66.

Renaud, M., F. Maquestiaux, S. Joncas, M. J. Kergoat, and L. Bherer. "The Effect of Three Months of Aerobic Training on Response Preparation in Older Adults." *Frontiers in Aging Neuroscience* 2 (2010): 148.

Shah, R. C., A. S. Buchman, R. S. Wilson, S. E. Leurgans, and D. A. Bennett. "Hemoglobin Level in Older Persons and Incident Alzheimer Disease: Prospective Cohort Analysis." *Neurology* 77, no. 3 (2011): 219–26.

Song, X., A. Mitnitski, and K. Rockwood. "Nontraditional Risk Factors Combine to Predict Alzheimer Disease and Dementia." *Neurology* 77, no. 3 (2011): 227–34.

CHAPTER 10

For more on wisdom with age and the potential contribution of older adults to community:

Baltes, P. *Wisdom as Orchestration of Mind and Virtue.* Max Planck Institute: Berlin, 2004. Available online at www.library.mpib-berlin. mpg.de/ft/pb/PB_Wisdom_2004.pdf

Cozolino, L. "The Healthy Aging Brain: Sustaining Attachment, Attaining Wisdom." *Norton Series on Interpersonal Neurobiology.* W. W. Norton & Company, 2008.

George, D. R., and P. J. Whitehouse. "Intergenerational Volunteering and Quality of Life for Persons with Mild-to-Moderate Dementia: Results from a 5-Month Intervention Study in the United States." *Journal of the American Geriatrics Society* 58, no. 4 (2010): 796–7.

Katz, A. M., Jr., L. Conant, T. S. Inuid, D. Baron, and D. Bor. "A Council of Elders: Creating a Multi-Voiced Dialogue in a Community of Care." *Social Science and Medicine* 50 (2000): 851–60.

For more on how Baycrest expanded the limits of care to create a Day Program for patients with frontotemporal dementia:

Grinberg, A., J. Lagunoff, D. Phillips, B. Stern, M. Goodman, T. W. Chow. "Multidisciplinary Design and Implementation of a Day Program Specialized for the Frontotemporal Dementias." *American Journal of Alzheimer's Disease and Other Disorders* 22, no. 6 (2007): 499–506.

For encouragement to engage and integrate:

Foresight and the new economics foundation. www.neweconomics. org/projects/five-ways-well-being

Fratiglioni, L., H. X. Wang, K. Ericsson, M. Maytan, and B. Winblad. "Influence of Social Network on Occurrence of Dementia: A Community-Based Longitudinal Study." *Lancet* 355, no. 9212 (2000): 1315–9.

CHAPTER 11

Nichols, K. R. *The Unspoken Gift* [forthcoming], see katherinenichols.com.

CHAPTER 12

For information on GPS or other systems for tracking patients who wander:

www.srs-mcmaster.ca/Portals/20/pdf/LTP_report.pdf and www.srs-mcmaster.ca/Portals/20/pdf/Locating_Technology_Tip_List.pdf

For more on management of responsive behaviors:

research.baycrest.org/chow-lab for interview with Dr. Dmytro Rewilak and the worksheet for caregivers.

For more on the consolidation function of sleep for learning, see work by Dan Margoliash of the University of Chicago: margoliashlab.uchicago.edu/publications

For more information on the Baycrest Frontotemporal Dementia Day Program, see citation in notes for Chapter 10.

The author's website for children who have parents with early-onset frontotemporal dementia:

www.lifeandminds.ca/whendementiaisinthehouse
and accompanying article:

Nichols, K. R., et al. "When Dementia Is in the House: Needs Assessment Survey for Young Caregivers." *Canadian Journal of Neurological Science.* 40, no. 1 (2013). [in press].

An activity book to educate younger children aged 5–9 years is available for free download at research.baycrest.org/chow-lab

For more on the amyloid theory of causation in Alzheimer's disease:
Cummings, J. L. "Alzheimer's Disease: Clinical Trials and the Amyloid Hypothesis." *Annals of the Academy of Medicine Singapore* 40, no. 7 (2011): 304–3.
Wang, A., P. Das, R. C. Switzer, 3rd, T. E. Golde, and J. L. Jankowsky. "Robust Amyloid Clearance in a Mouse Model of Alzheimer's Disease Provides Novel Insights into the Mechanism of Amyloid-Beta Immunotherapy." *Journal of Neuroscience* 31, no. 11 (2011): 4124–36.

CHAPTER 13

For more about Rick Morimoto's lab:
www.cgm.northwestern.edu/cgm/Faculty-Research/Faculty/Richard-Morimoto

For the prion story within Alzheimer's disease:
Stöhr J., et al. "Purified and Synthetic Alzheimer's Amyloid Beta (Aβ) Prions." *Proceedings of the National Academy of Science USA* 109, no. 27 (2012): 11025–30. Epub 2012 Jun 18.

For more on proving the involvement of prions in the spread of protein-opathy, see Neil Cashman of the University of British Columbia's work:
www.prionetcanada.ca/detail.aspx?menu=2&app=95&cat1=377&t-p=2&lk=no&title=Staff+Biographies#cashman

For more on getting the bouncers to work on discouraging abnormal protein aggregation:
Gillette-Guyonnet, S., and B. Vellas. "Caloric Restriction and Brain Function." *Current Opinion in Clinical Nutrition and Metabolic Care* 11, no. 6 (2008): 686–92.
Golde, T. E., L. S. Schneider, and E. H. Koo. "Anti-Abeta Therapeutics in Alzheimer's Disease: The Need for a Paradigm Shift." *Neuron* 69, no. 2 (2011): 203–13.

For a comprehensive, well-organized review of tried-and-untrue therapies:

Lauterback, E. C., and M. F. Mendez. "Psychopharmacologic Neuro-protection in Neurodegenerative Diseases, Part III: Criteria-Based Assessment: A Report of the ANPA Committee on Research." *Journal of Neuropsychology and Clinical Neuroscience* 23 (2011): 242–60.

For more on Rosa Rademakers's work: mayoresearch.mayo.edu/mayo/research/Staff/Rademakers_R8.cfm.

For more on anti-tau therapies:

Gong, C. X., I. Grundke-Iqbal, and K. Iqbal. "Targeting Tau Protein in Alzheimer's Disease." *Drugs Aging* 27, no. 5 (2010): 351–65.

Virginia Lee and John Trojanowski at the University of Pennsylvania Center for Neurodegenerative Disease Research: www.med.upenn.edu/cndr.

For more on GSK-3a inhibition:

Gandy, S. and B. Wustman. "New Pathway Links Gamma-Secretase to Inflammation and Memory While Sparing Notch [Editorial]." *Annals of Neurology* 69, no. 1 (2010): 5–7.

Pre-clinical trials are an important starting point for the development of drugs. The non-human subjects of those experiments are not always rats!

Karen Ashe began in the 1990s to create transgenic mice. These animals have been genetically tinkered with to replicate the brain changes of dementia. Focusing on Alzheimer's disease, Ashe began with "knock-out" transgenic mice, which were engineered to show what mayhem follows deletion of a key factor for suppressing proteinopathy. More recently there are "knock-in" mice, into which a threatening gene can be introduced to the mouse's original DNA to observe what transpires at the molecular level. For a while, we had transgenic mice with either tangles or plaques, neither of which completely reproduces an Alzheimer's brain, but now we have a mouse that has it all, in a bad way. This mouse with three insults to the brain (amyloid plaques, tangles, and impaired plasticity) more closely approximates the process of Alzheimer's disease in humans. www.neurosci.umn.edu/faculty/hsiao.html

Flies, mice, and worms are the most common animal models that help us determine when proteinopathy begins. Neuroscientist George Jackson (www.utmb.edu/ncb/faculty/GeorgeJackson/GeorgeR Jackson.asp) monitors the consequences of genetic mutations related to neurodegenerative diseases when those mutations are inserted into fruit flies (*Drosophila*). The mutation gets the flies to produce the abnormal proteins implicated in dementia processes. When we try to detect symptoms of dementia in people, we have to interview them or test their cognition. But that can't be done with a fly, and fruit flies are minuscule compared with the common housefly, so George rigged the experimental fruit flies to manifest grotesque abnormalities on the surfaces of their eyes to signal that inserted mutations had taken hold in the nervous system. He has created monsters that not even a pre-med student would mistake for normal. These relatively inexpensive animal models are then used to test interventions against the unwanted accumulation of the misfolded, sticky protein. If any candidate treatment were to work, his post-mutation monster would revert to normally smooth eyes again. Even worms have been important models for showing how the unwanted, misfolded protein might be earlier detected within the cell so that it can be defused before it becomes a threat to the neuron. The team at UCSF has been working on a worm model for frontotemporal dementia. Jiao, J., et al. "Microrna-29b Regulates the Expression Level of Human Progranulin, a Secreted Glycoprotein Implicated in Frontotemporal Dementia." *Public Library of Science One* 5, no. 5 (2010): e10551.

Given the high costs of running clinical trials in human subjects, testing new treatments sensibly starts with animal models ... even a non-animal, living model, like yeast!

The advantage of switching from rodents to yeast is that the more simple the organism, the less expensive conducting tests on it is. As well, the non-human models have shorter life cycles, which means that results may not take as long to observe and report. [Treusch S., et al. "Functional Links Between Aβ Toxicity, Endocytic Trafficking, and Alzheimer's Disease Risk Factors in Yeast." *Science* 334 (6060) (2011): 1241–5.] The downside is that the researchers are trying to re-create the effects of dementia on a complex organ (the brain) in humans who have complex behaviors and cognitive functions.

For more on the author's open-label memantine trial for frontotemporal dementia:

Chow, T. W., et al. "An Open-Label Study of the Short-Term Effects of Memantine on FDG-PET in Frontotemporal Dementia." *Neuropsychiatric Disease and Treatment 7*, no. 1 (2011): 415–424.

Chow, T. W., et al. "FDG-PET in Semantic Dementia After 6 Months of Memantine: An Open-Label Study." *International Journal of Geriatric Psychiatry*, 2012. [Epub ahead of print].

CHAPTER 14

For stories about the effects of Hansen's disease on Hawai'ians:

Pi'ilani Ko'olau. *Kaluaikoolau*, as told to John G.M. Sheldon, 1906. Translated later by Helen N. Frazier as "The True Story of Kaluaikoolau, or Ko'olau the Leper." *Hawaiian Journal of History* 1987: 21. Fictionalized most recently by poet Merwin, W. S. *The Folding Cliffs: A Narrative of 19th-Century Hawaii*. Knopf, 2000.

Tayman, J. *The Colony*. Scribner, 2006.

APPENDIX 3

This appendix is the scoring system from Kivipelto M., et al. "Risk Score for the Prediction of Dementia Risk in 20 Years Among Middle Aged People: A Longitudinal, Population-Based Study." *Lancet Neurology* 5, no. 9 (2006): 735–41.

Another scale, for those who are already over age 70, is Barnes, D. E., et al. "Predicting Risk of Dementia in Older Adults. The Late-Life Dementia Risk Index." *Neurology* 73 (2009): 173–9.

GRATITUDE

Mucho mahalo to *kokua* Beverly Slopen, for her faith that I have a story to tell and for nurturing the process; to Diane Turbide at Penguin for midwifery of this book; to Rick and Jan, Russ and Charlotte Lesser for providing this amateur writer with garrets by the seashore; to Lynn Posluns for bringing me onto the Women of Baycrest launch team and thereby sparking the idea of entwining my story with Ah Quan's in this way; to Carol White of the Hawai'ian Mission Children's Society Library at Mission Houses in Honolulu; to Tracy Burgo, Diane Moses, and Linda Wong at the Board of Hawai'ian Water Supply, who helped me retrieve precious messages from Ah Quan for the family; and to Neil, William, and John Skinner on the homefront, who granted me the gift of time for book editing. May we all be safe, loved, happy, and healthy.

INDEX